This Book Belongs To:

____

____

____

Test Your Color

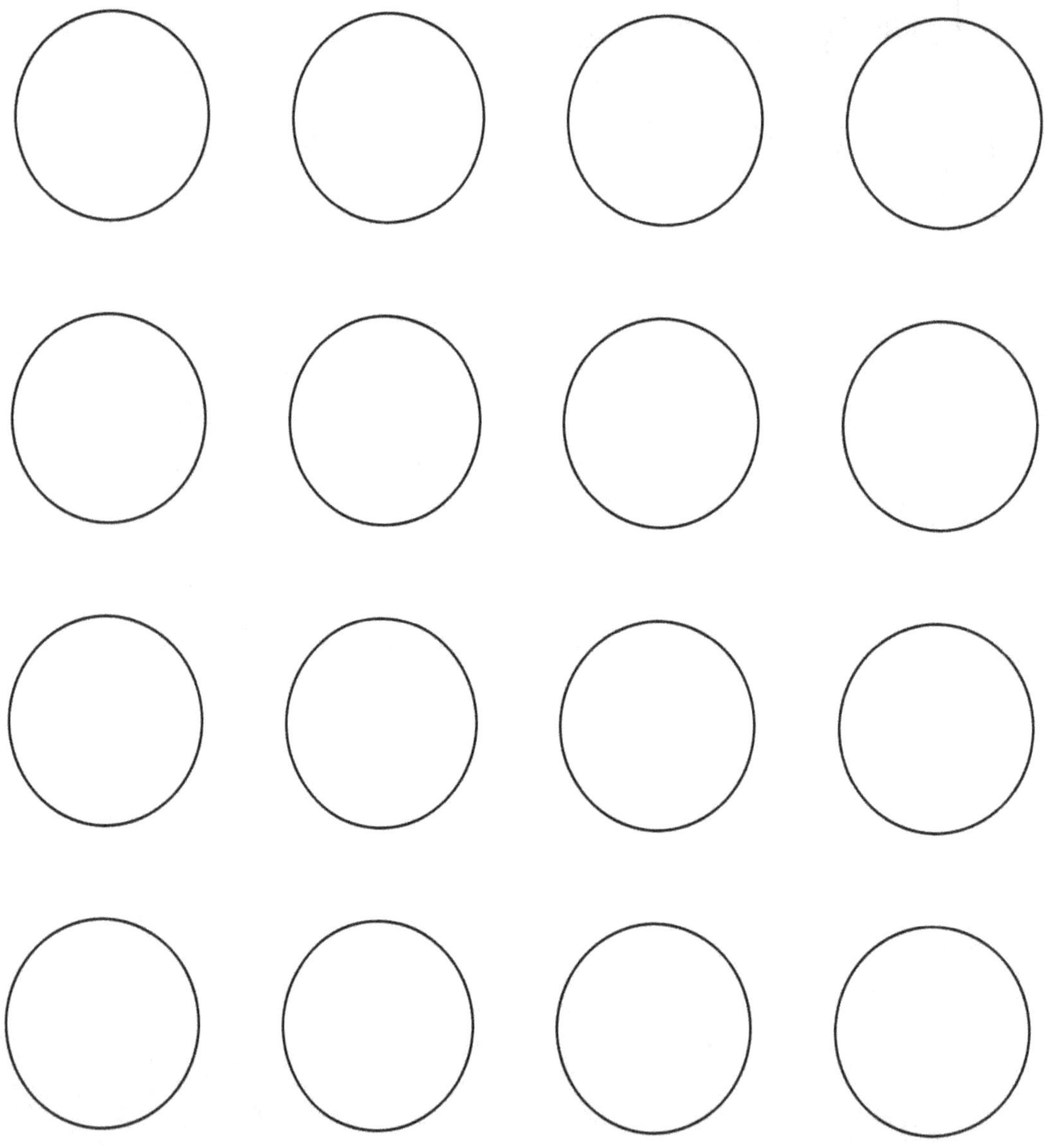

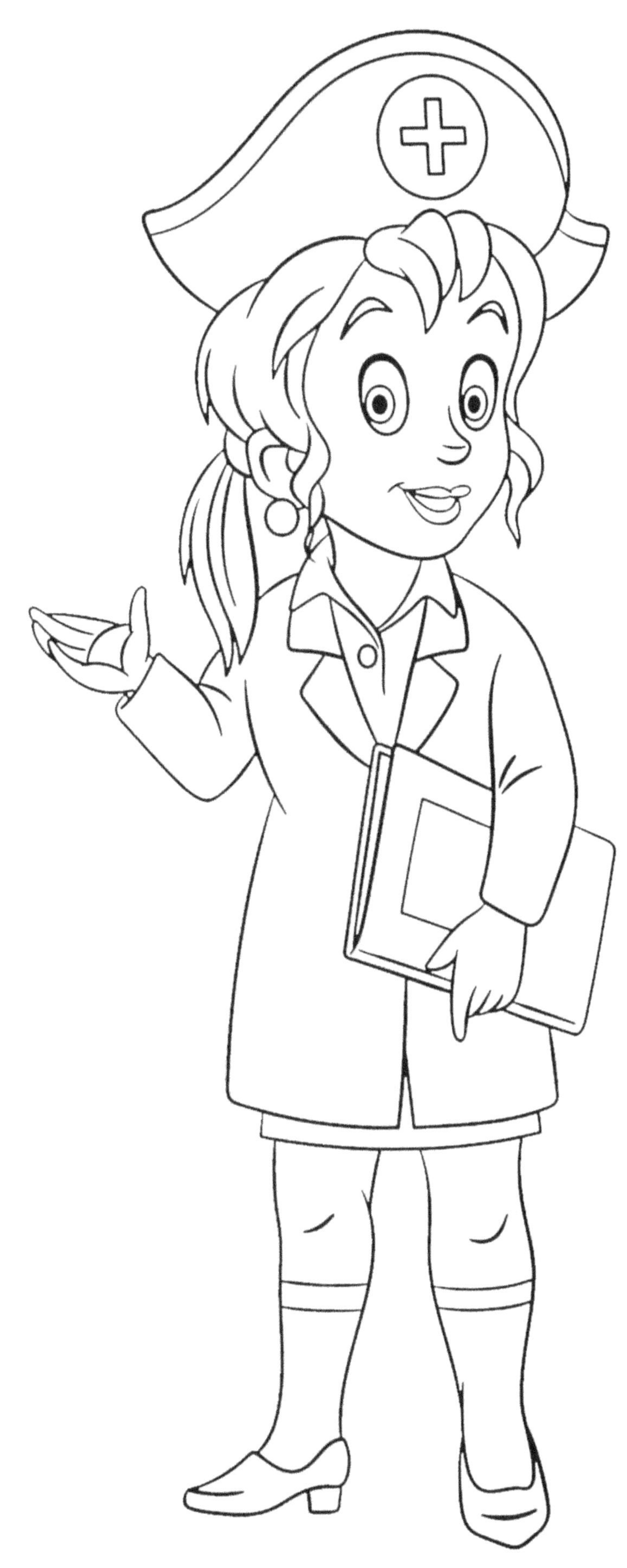

Test Your Color

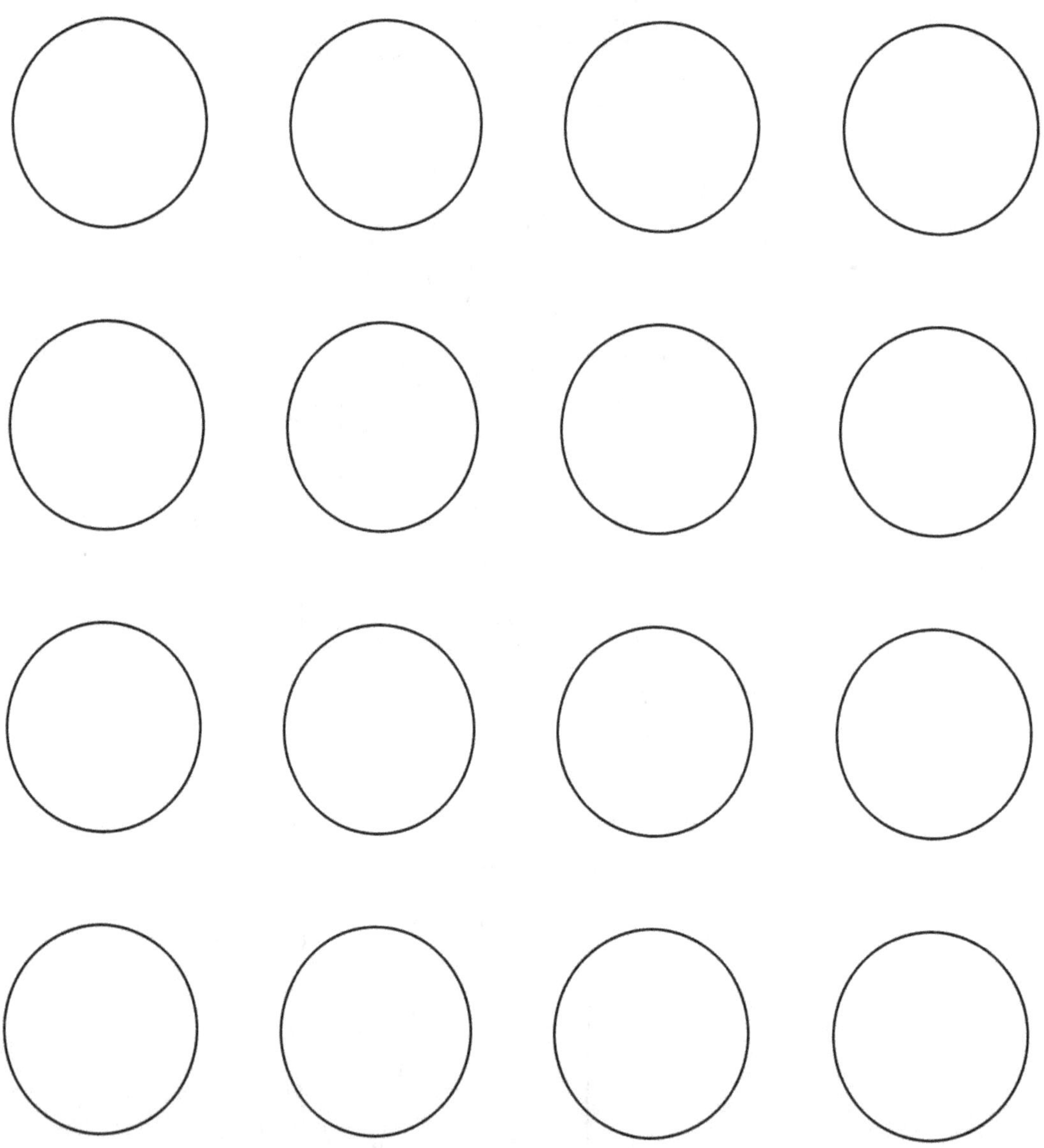

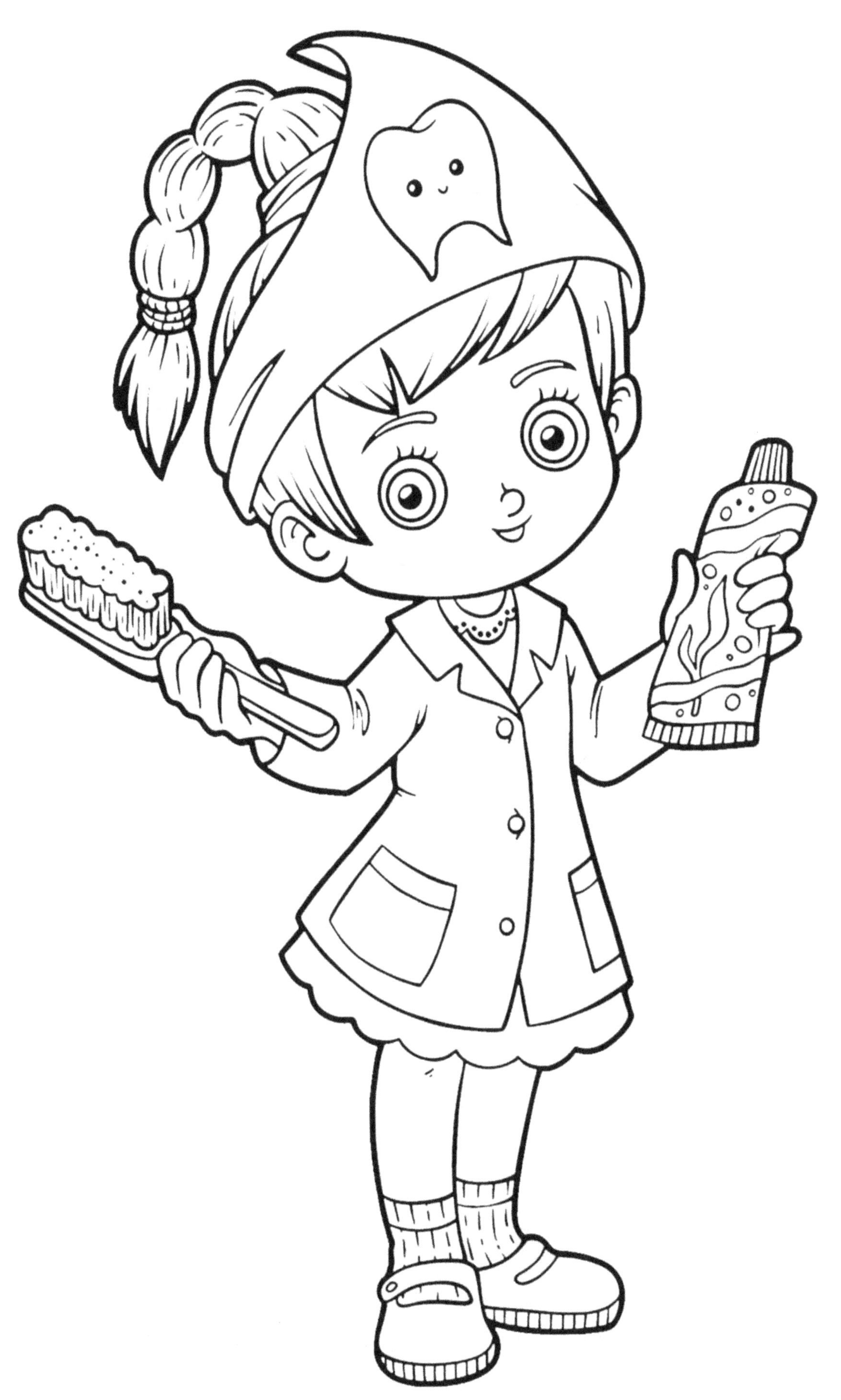

Test Your Color

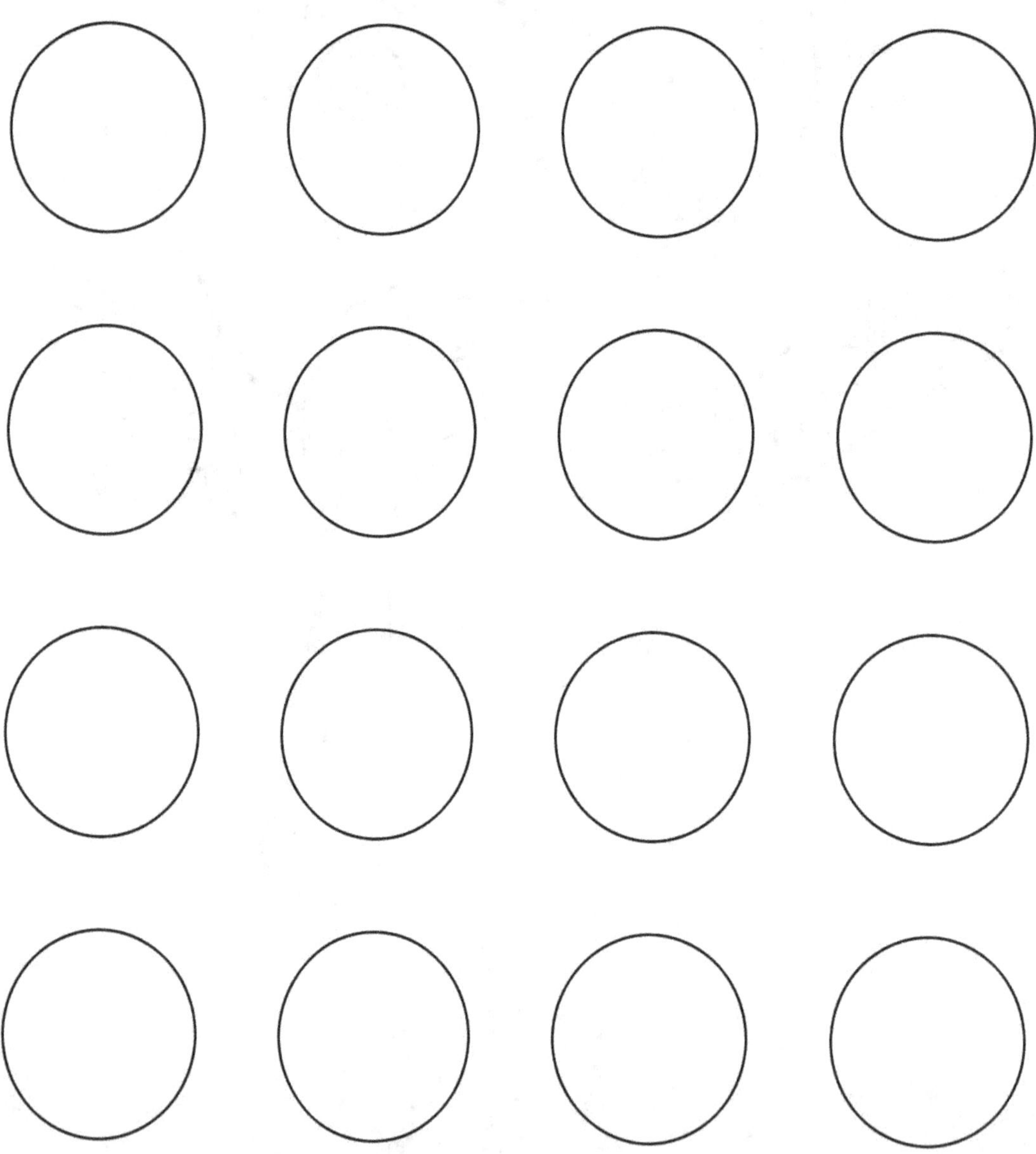

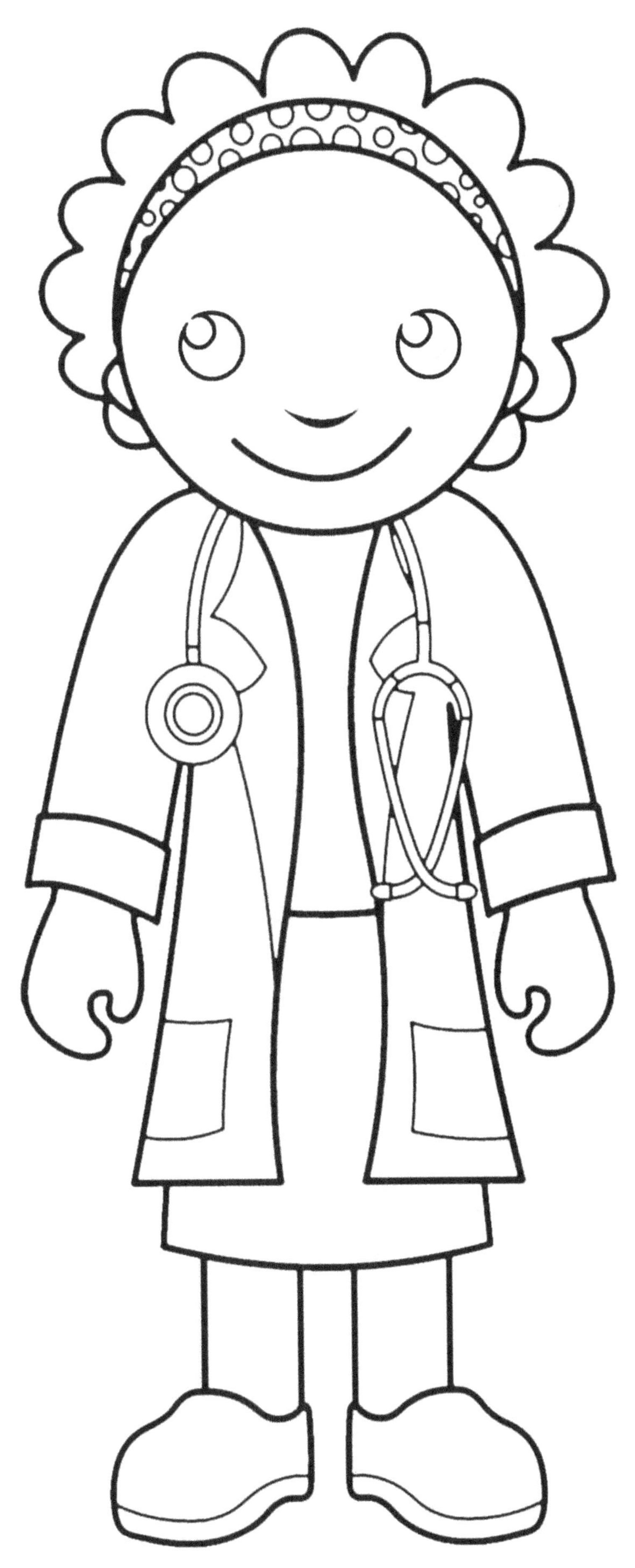

Test Your Color

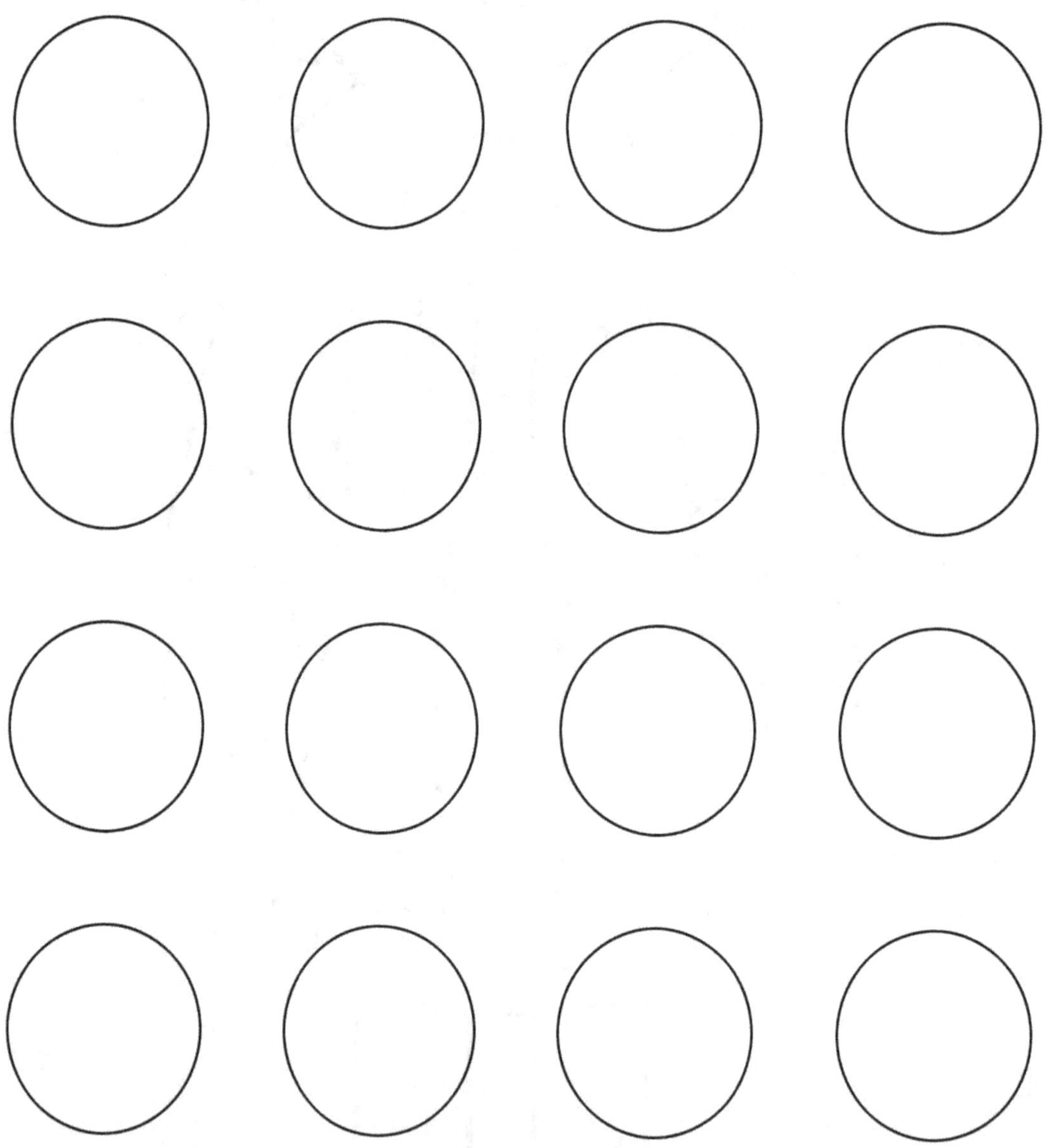

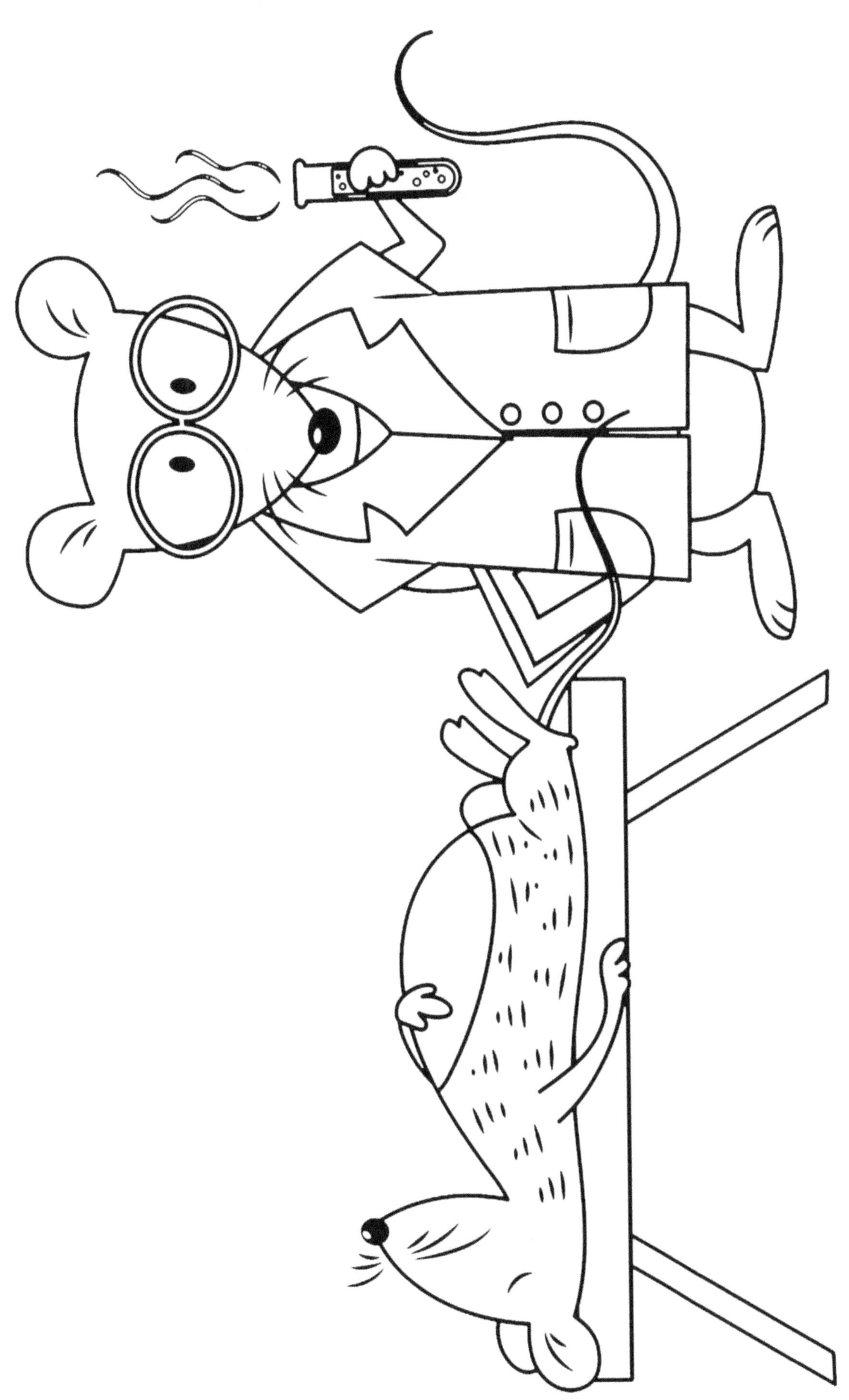

Test Your Color

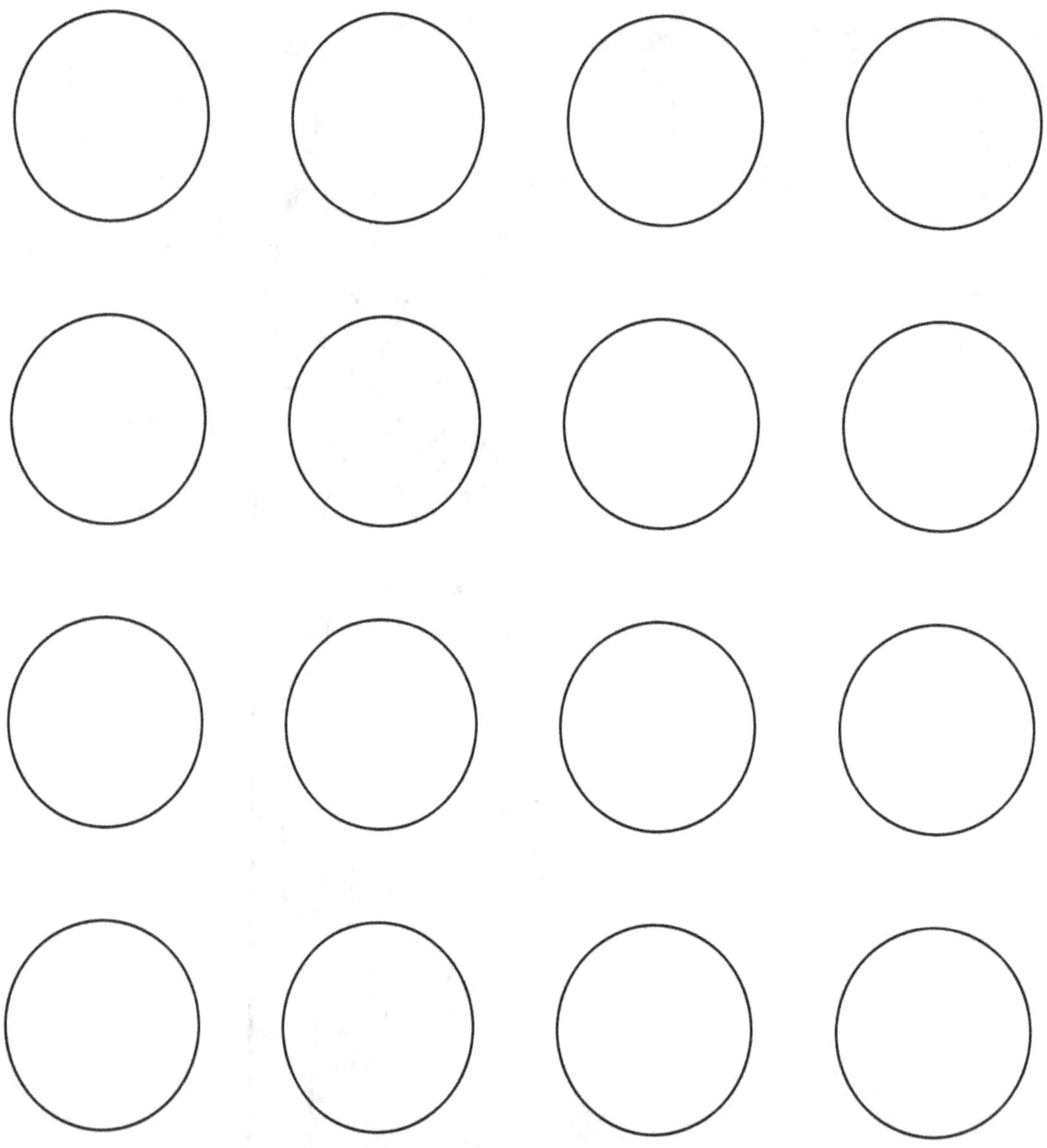

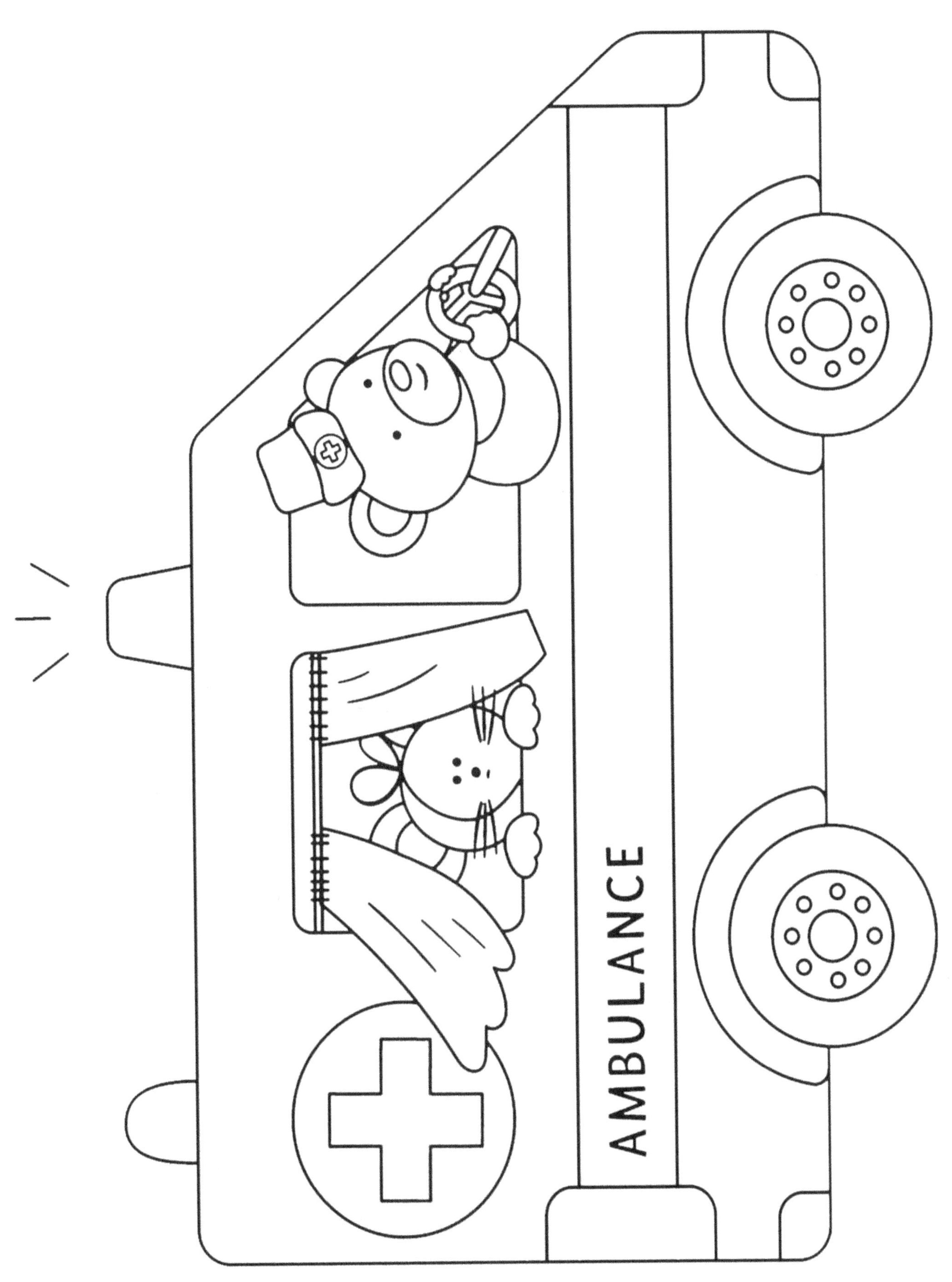
AMBULANCE

Test Your Color

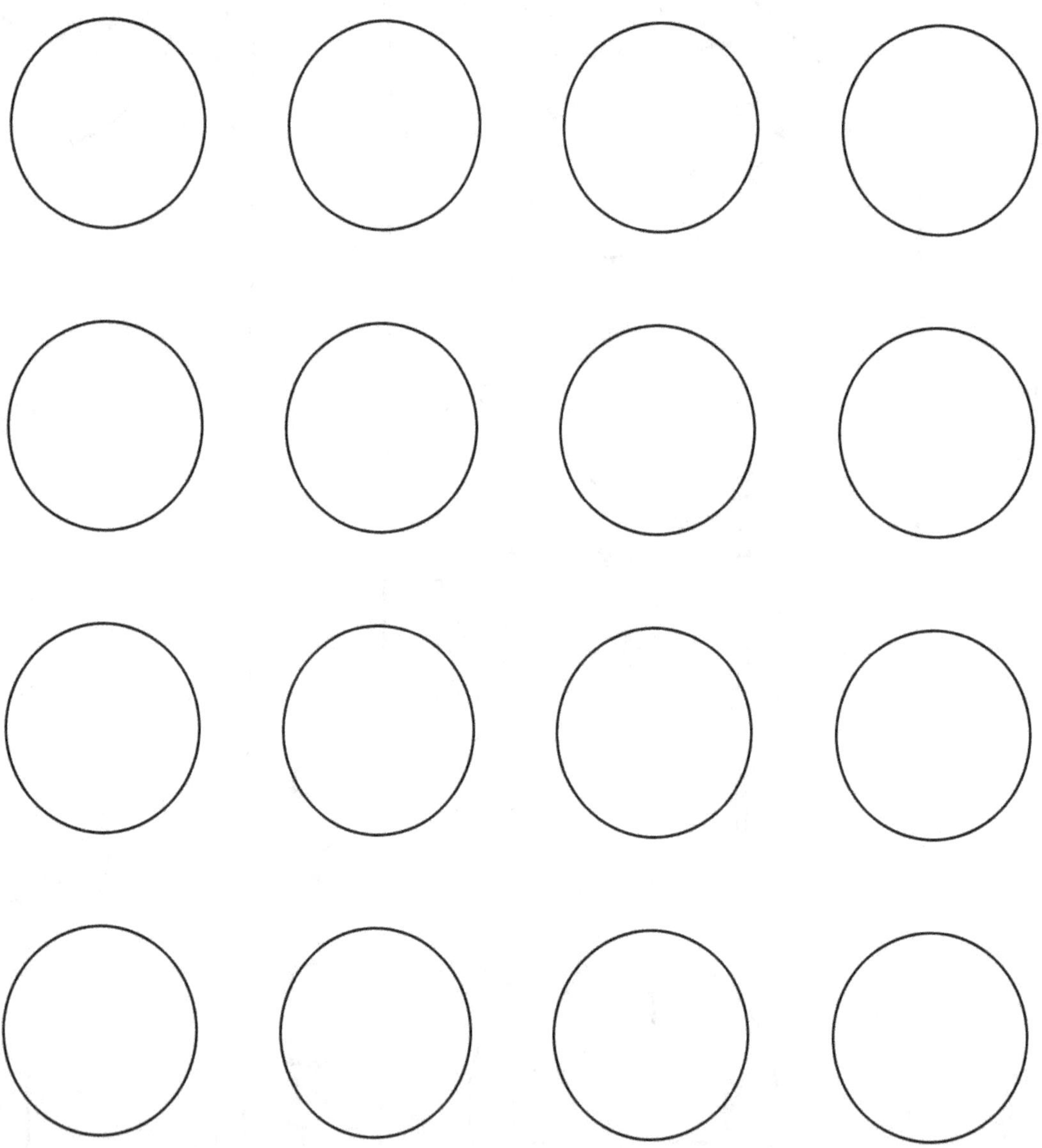

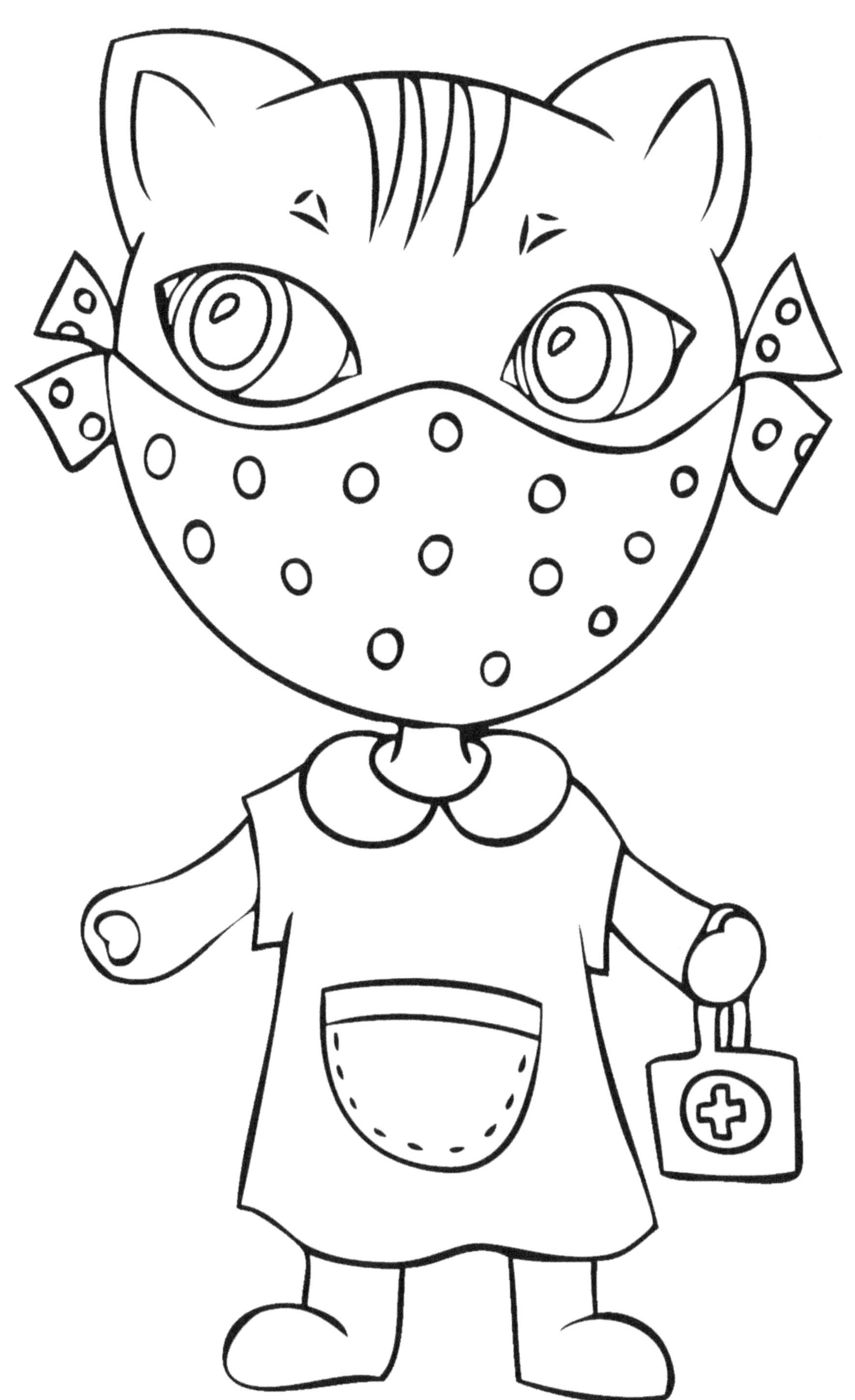

Test Your Color

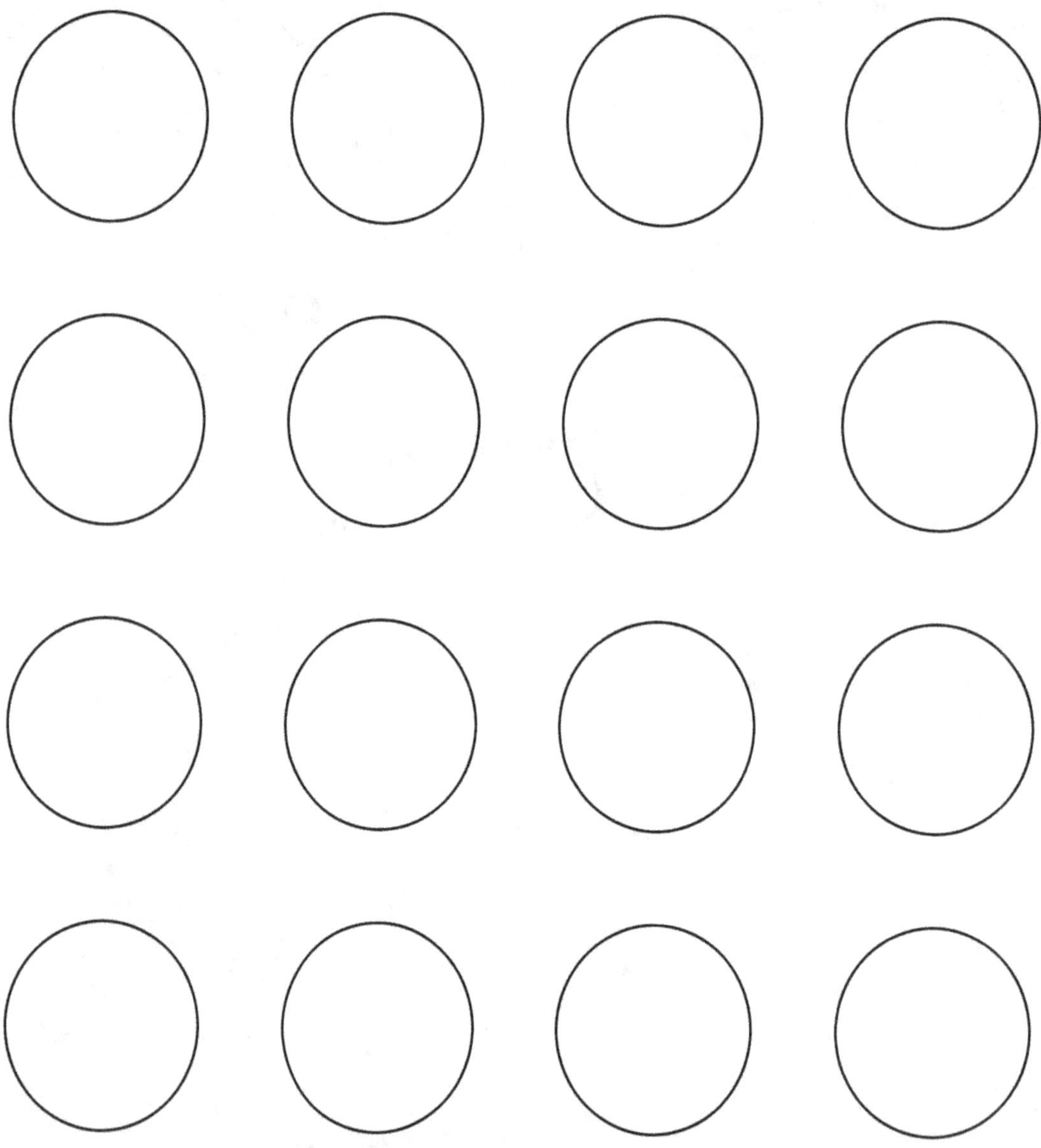

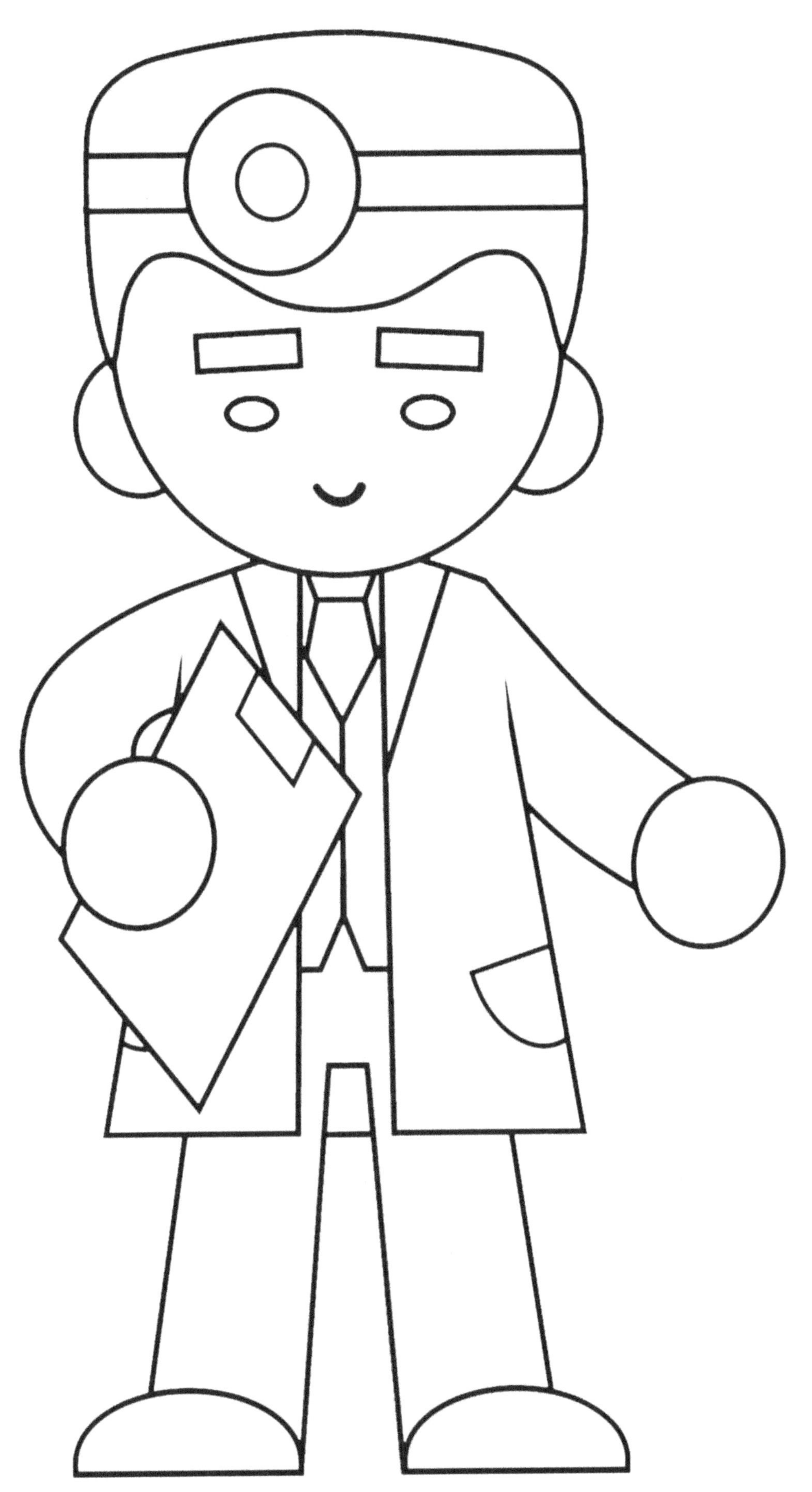

Test Your Color

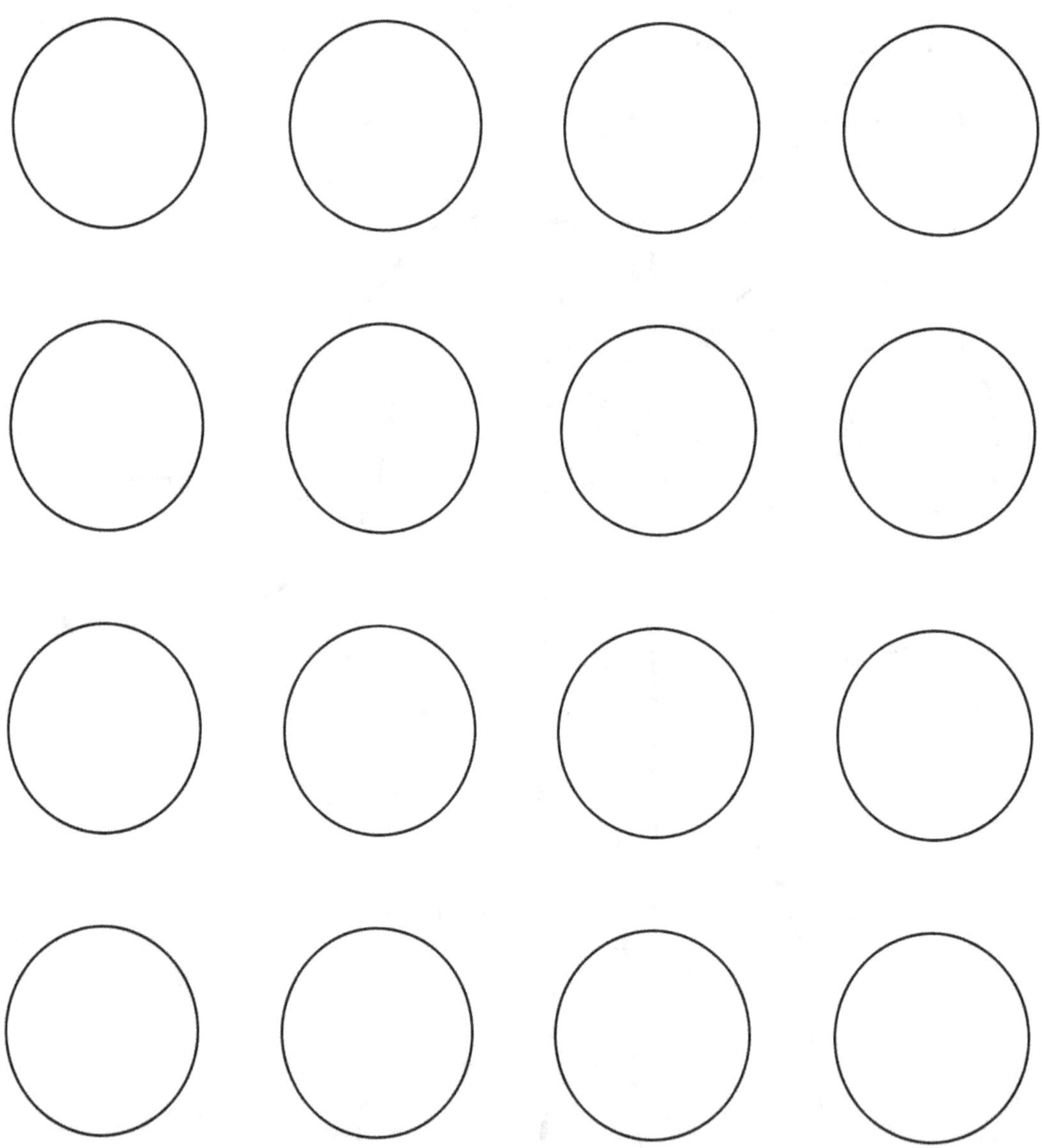

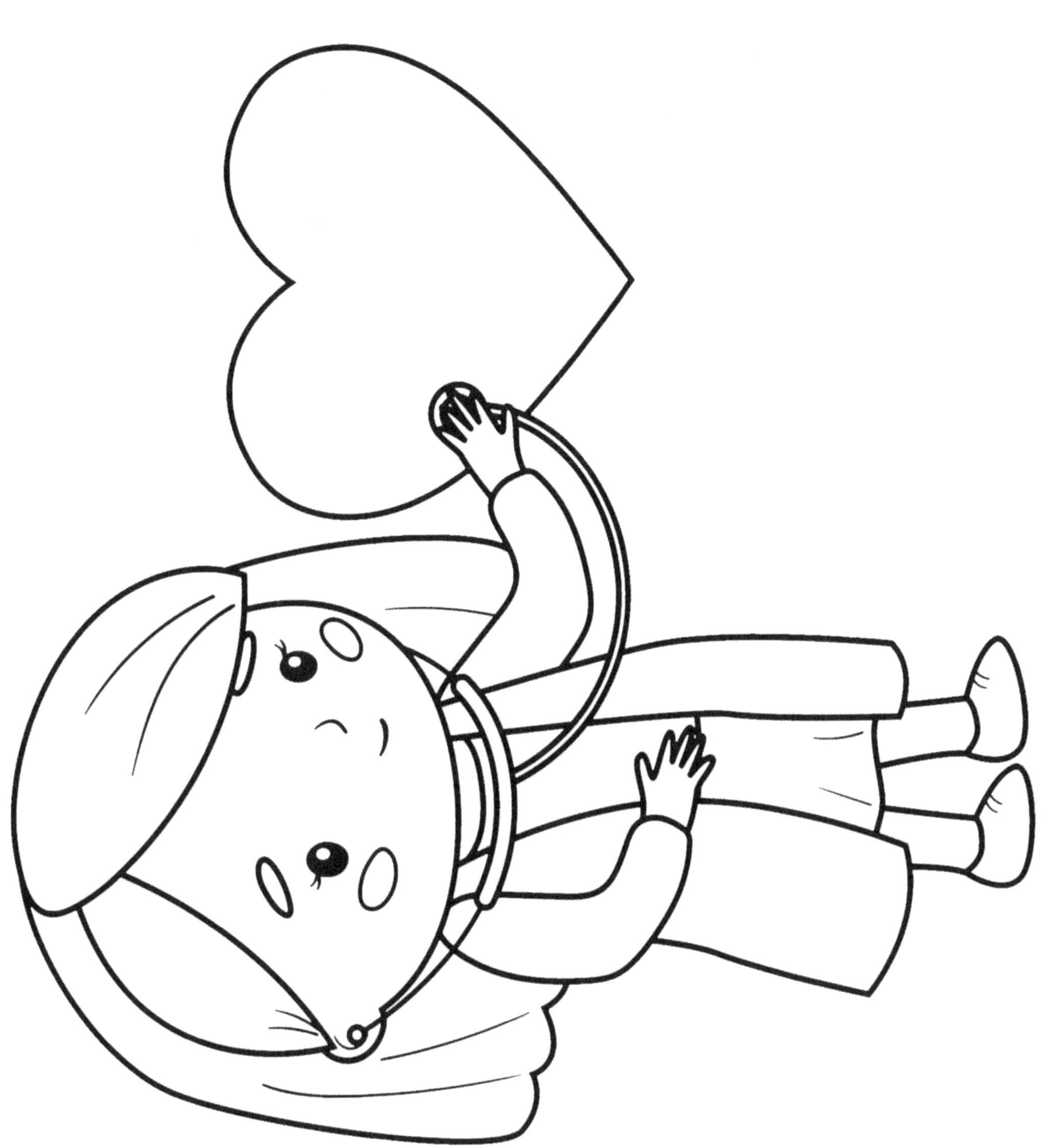

Test Your Color

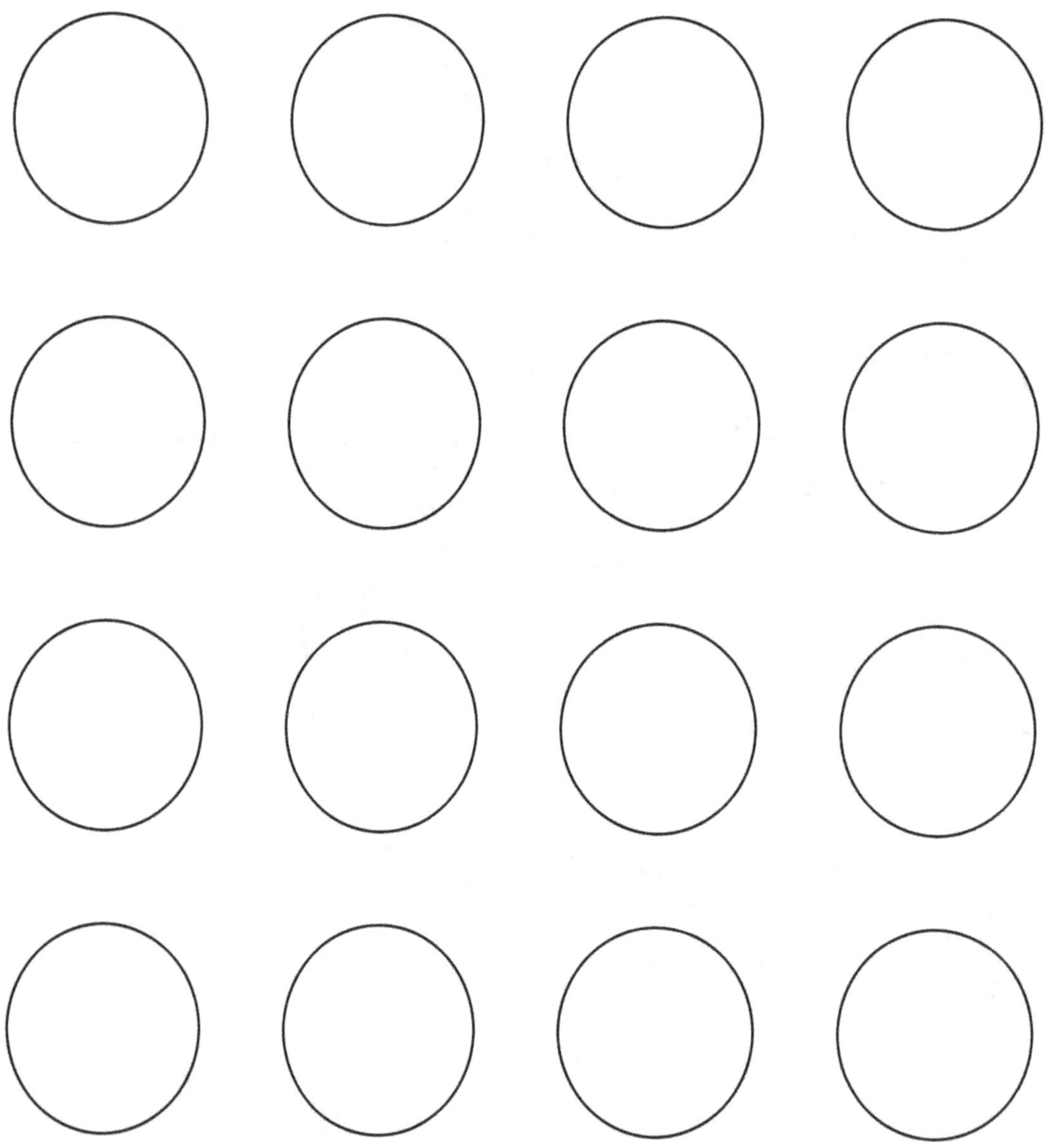

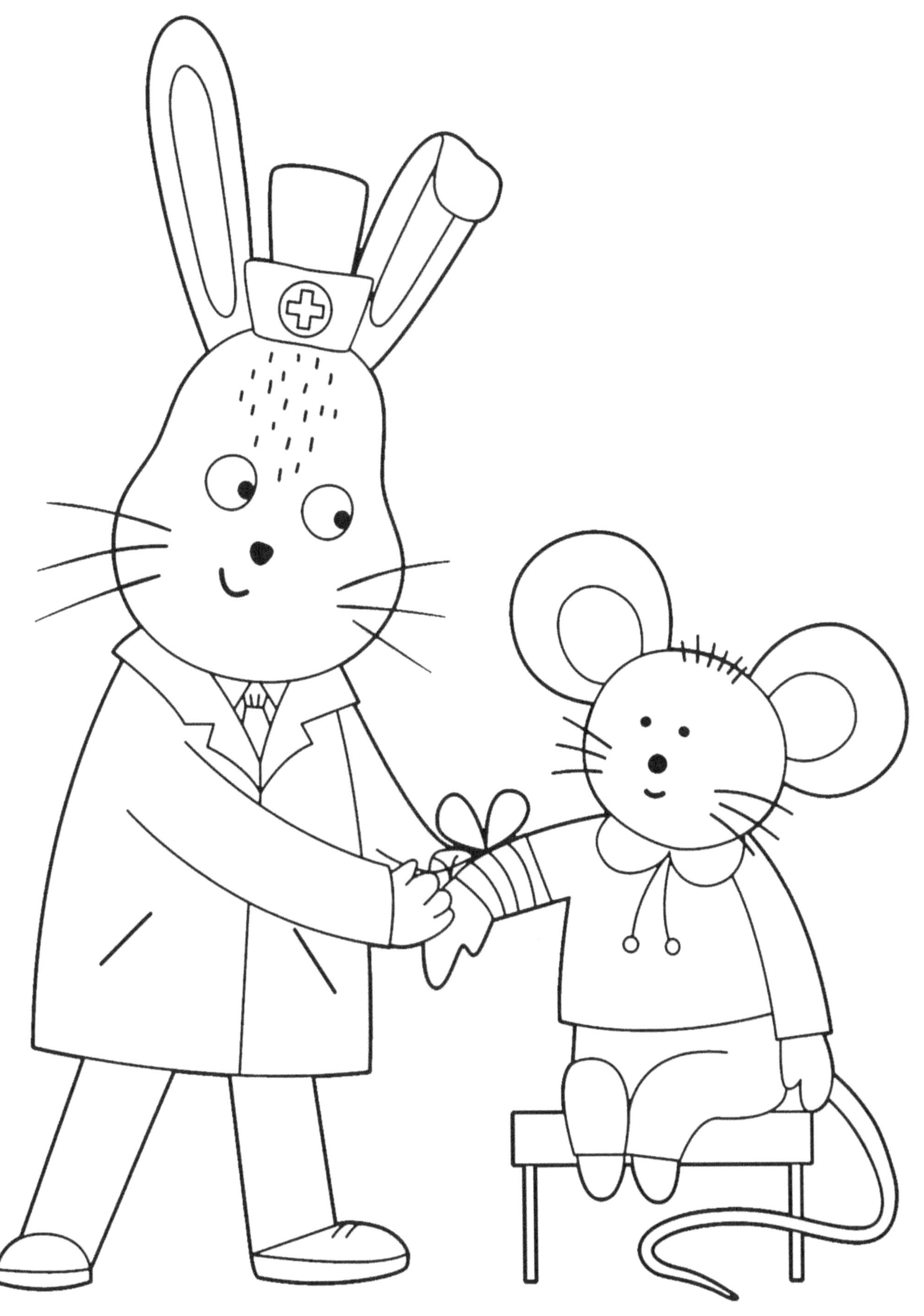

Test Your Color

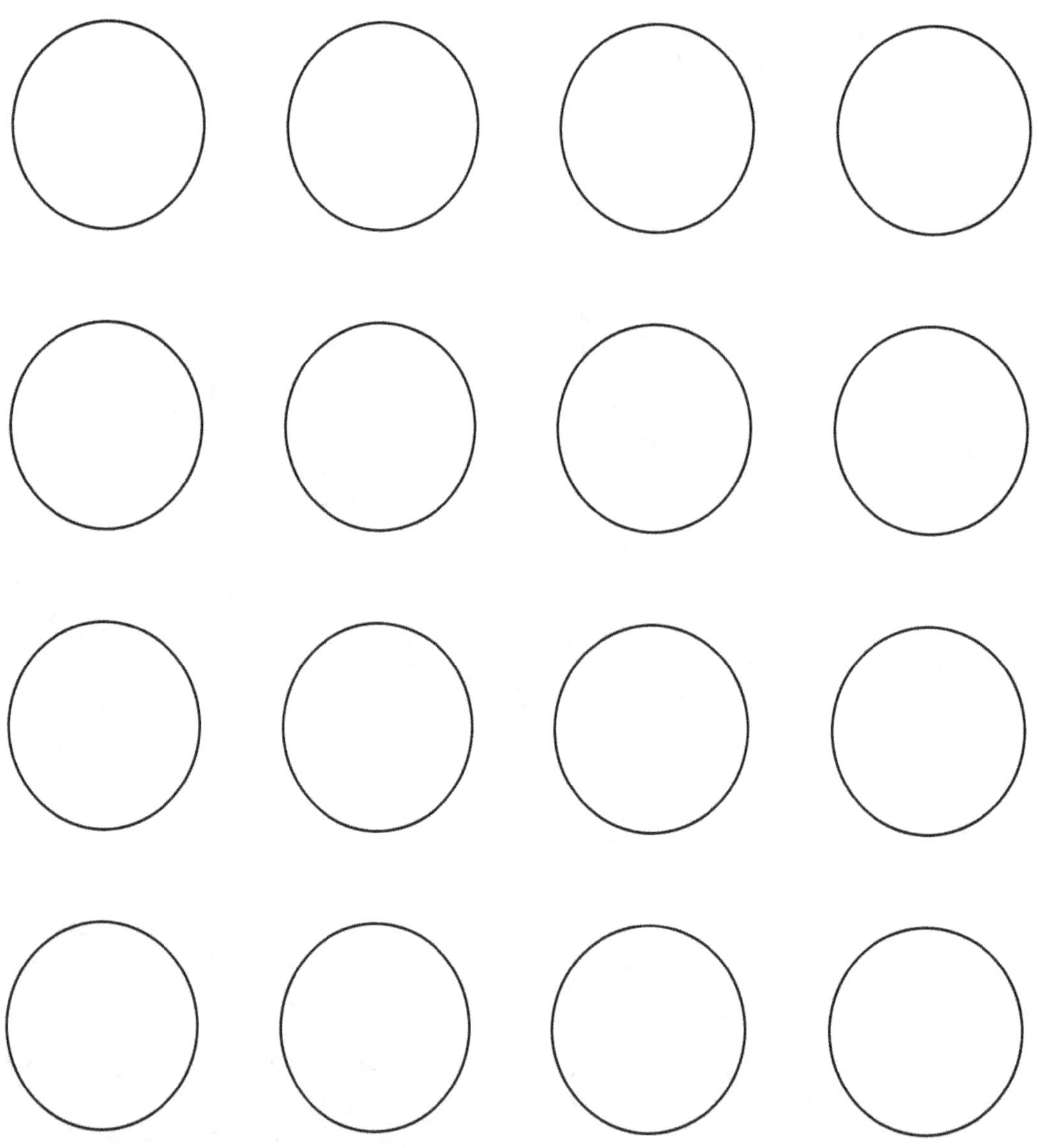

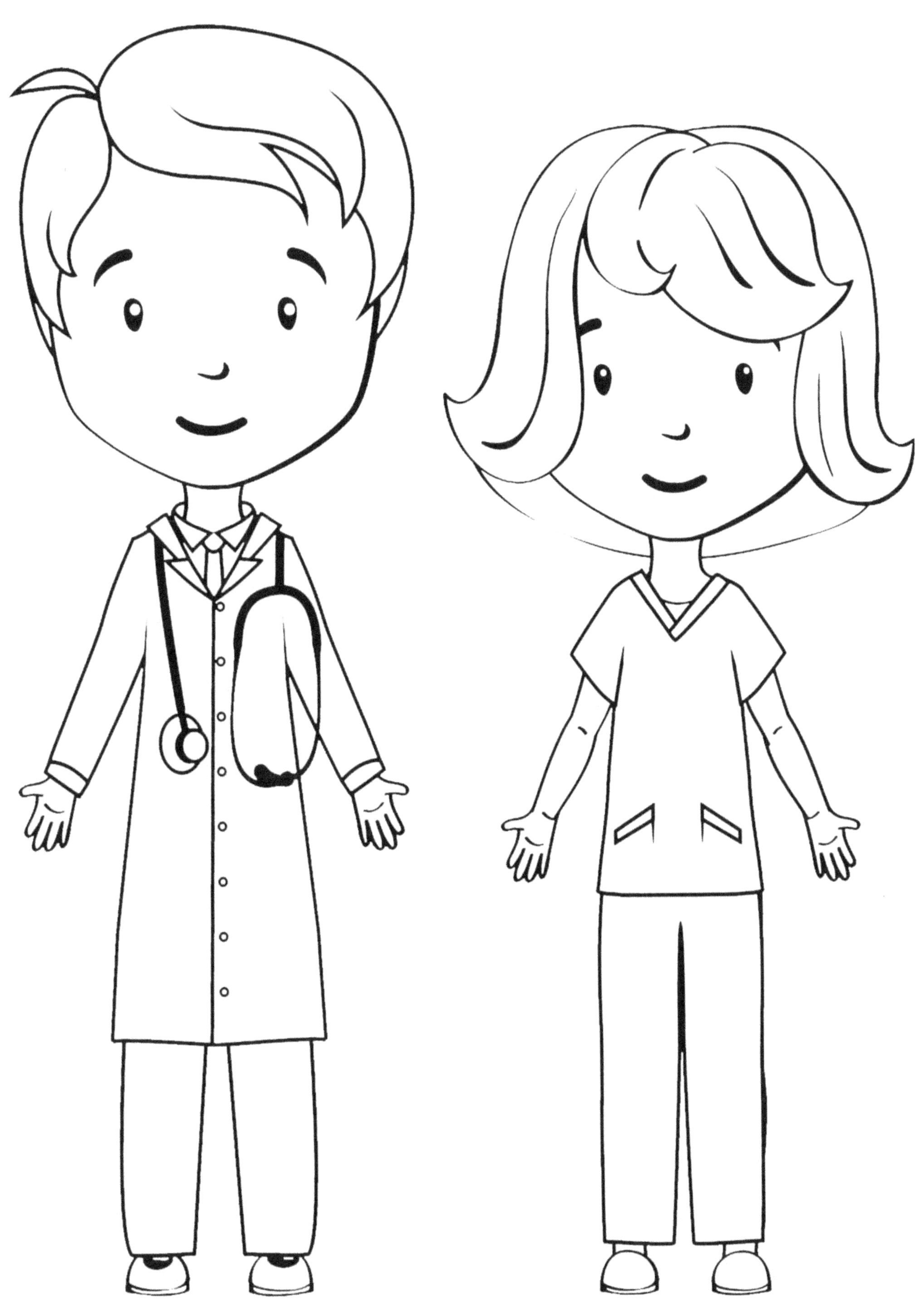

Test Your Color

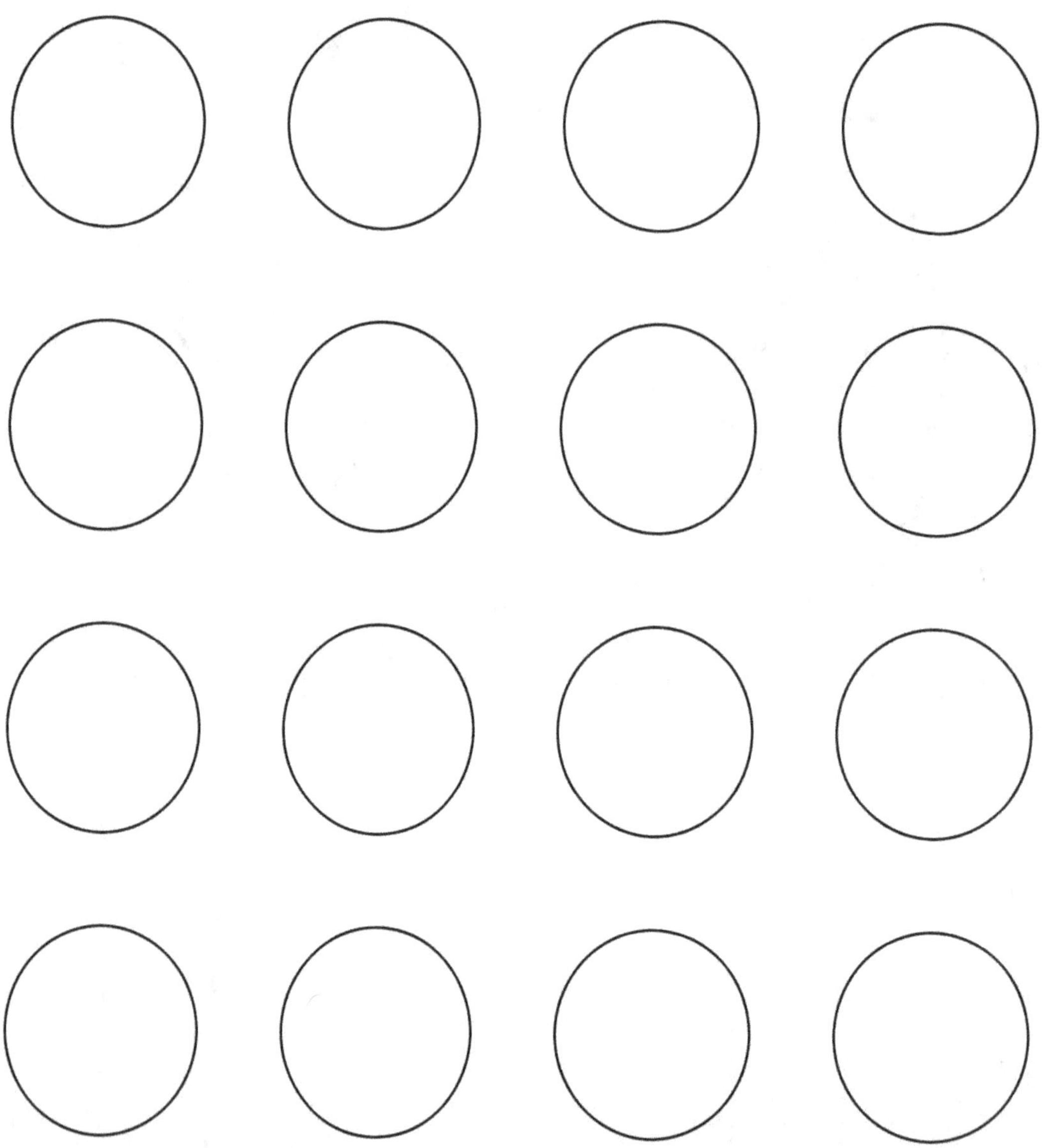

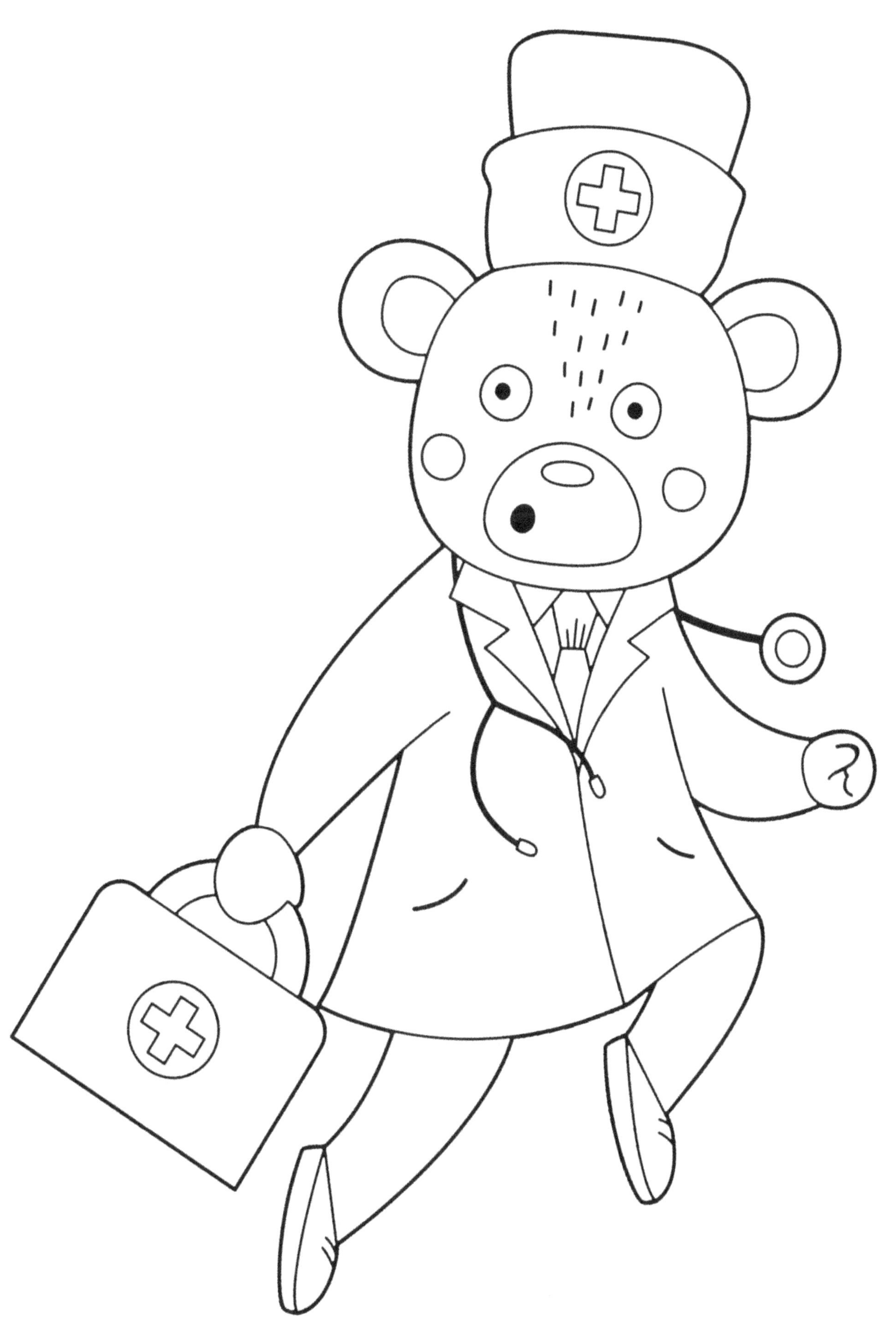

Test Your Color

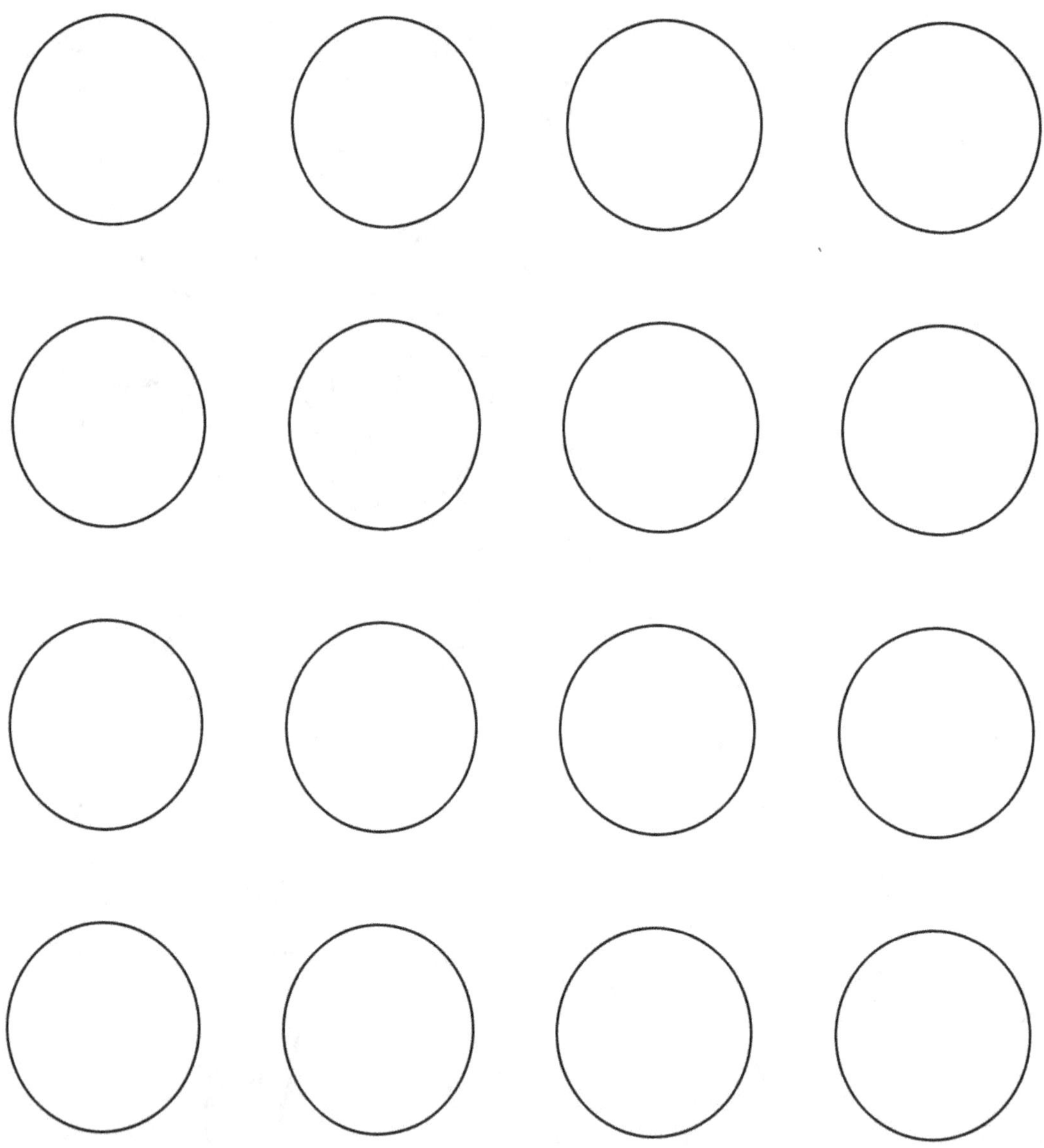

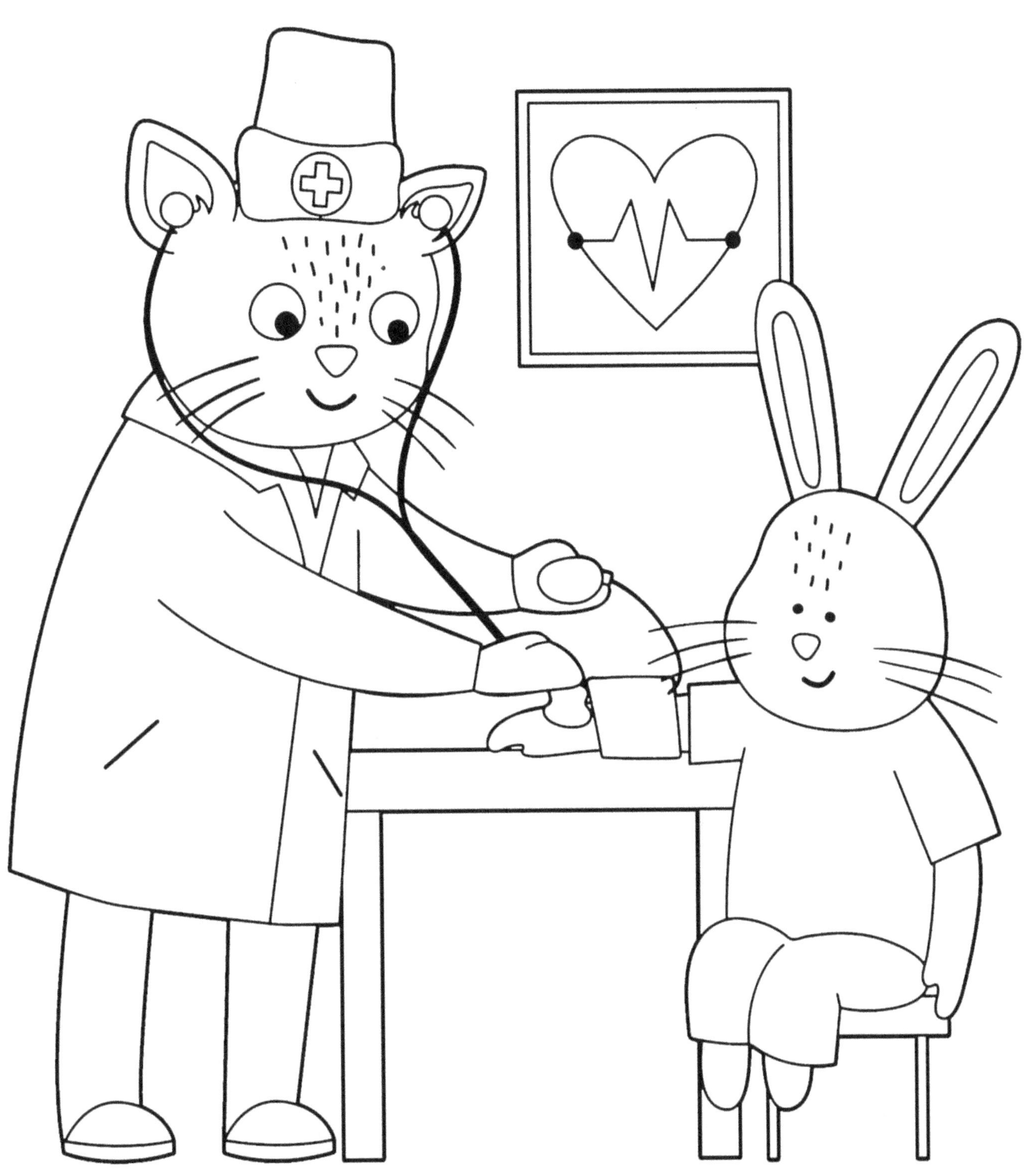

Test Your Color

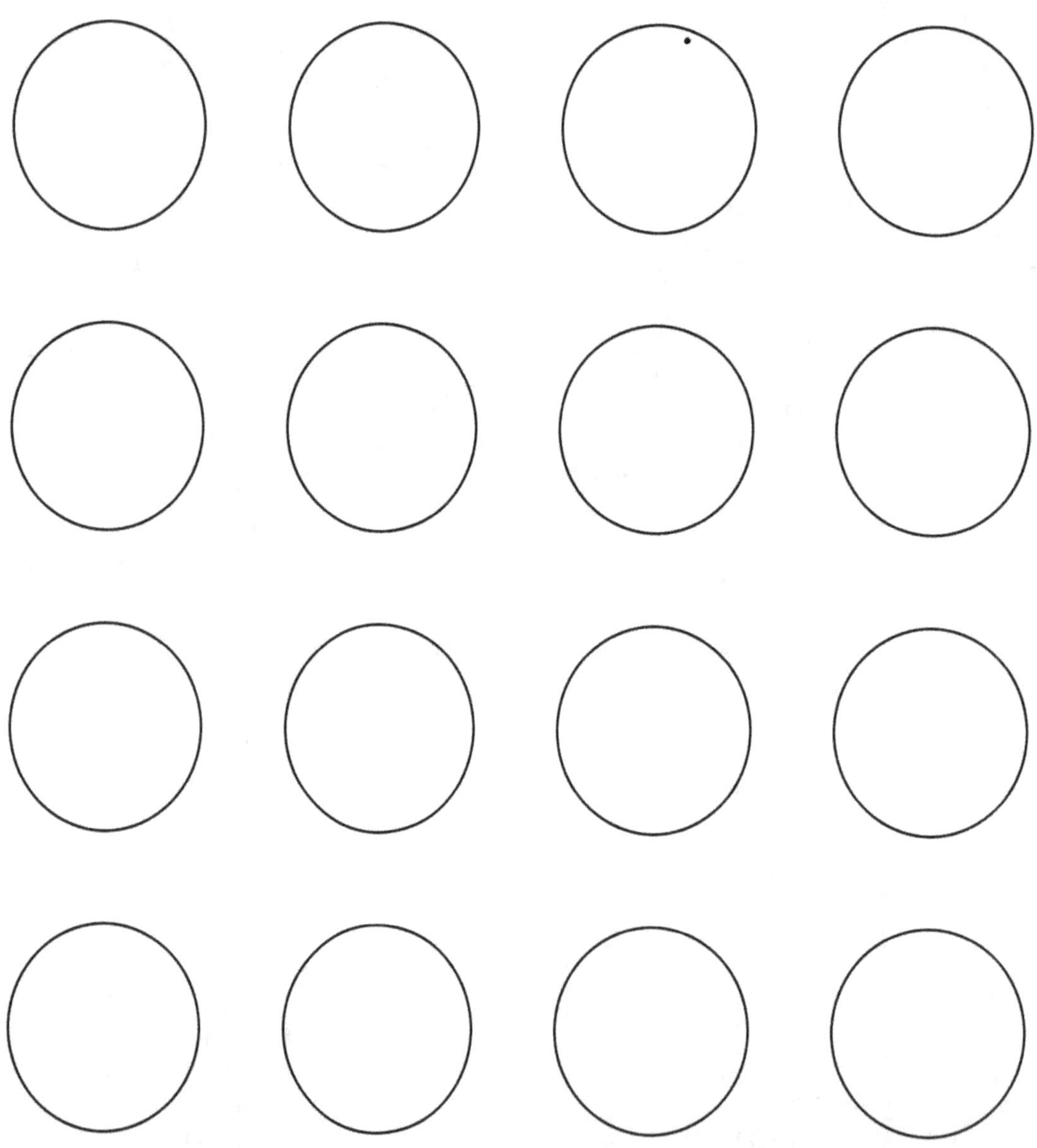

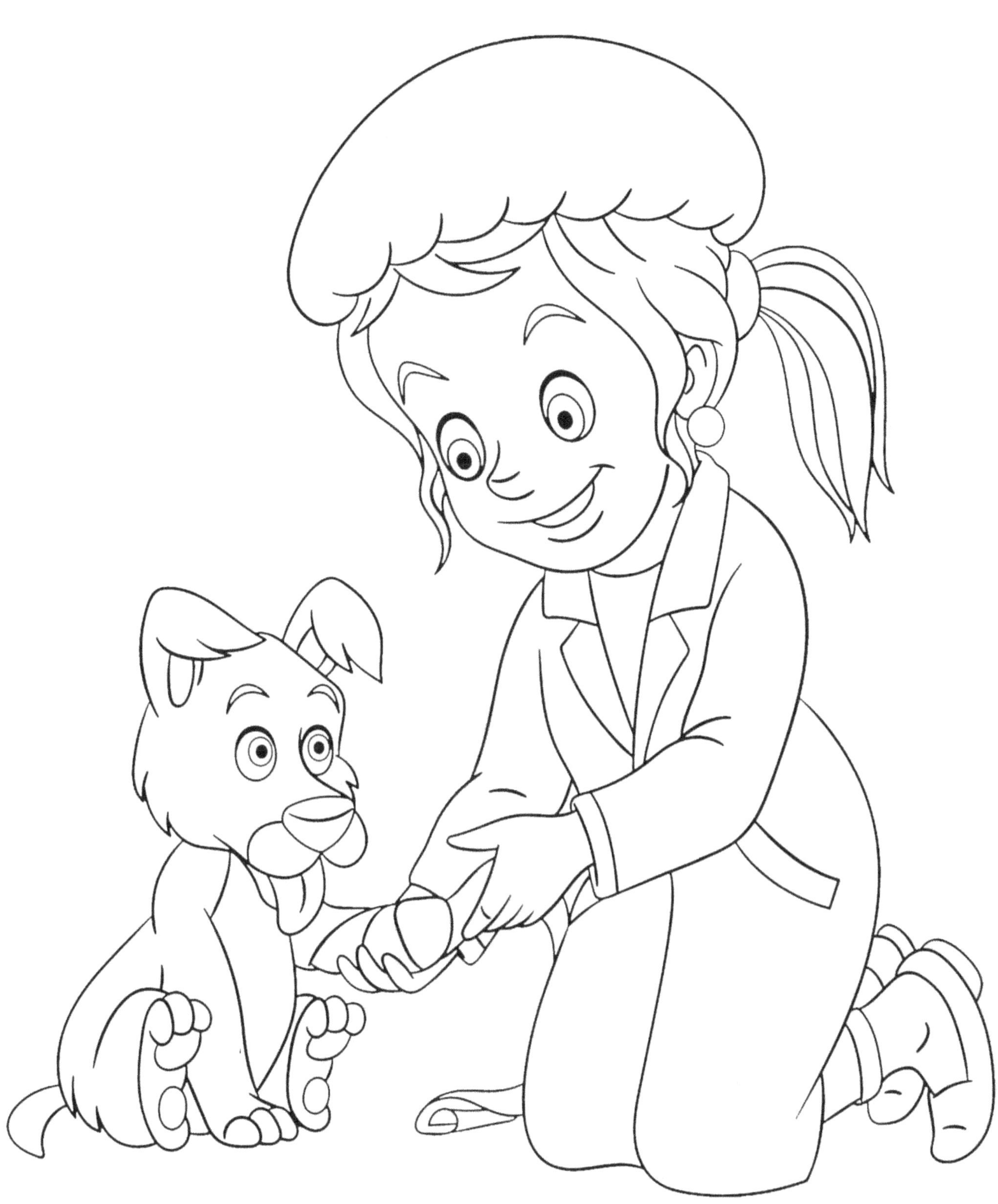

Test Your Color

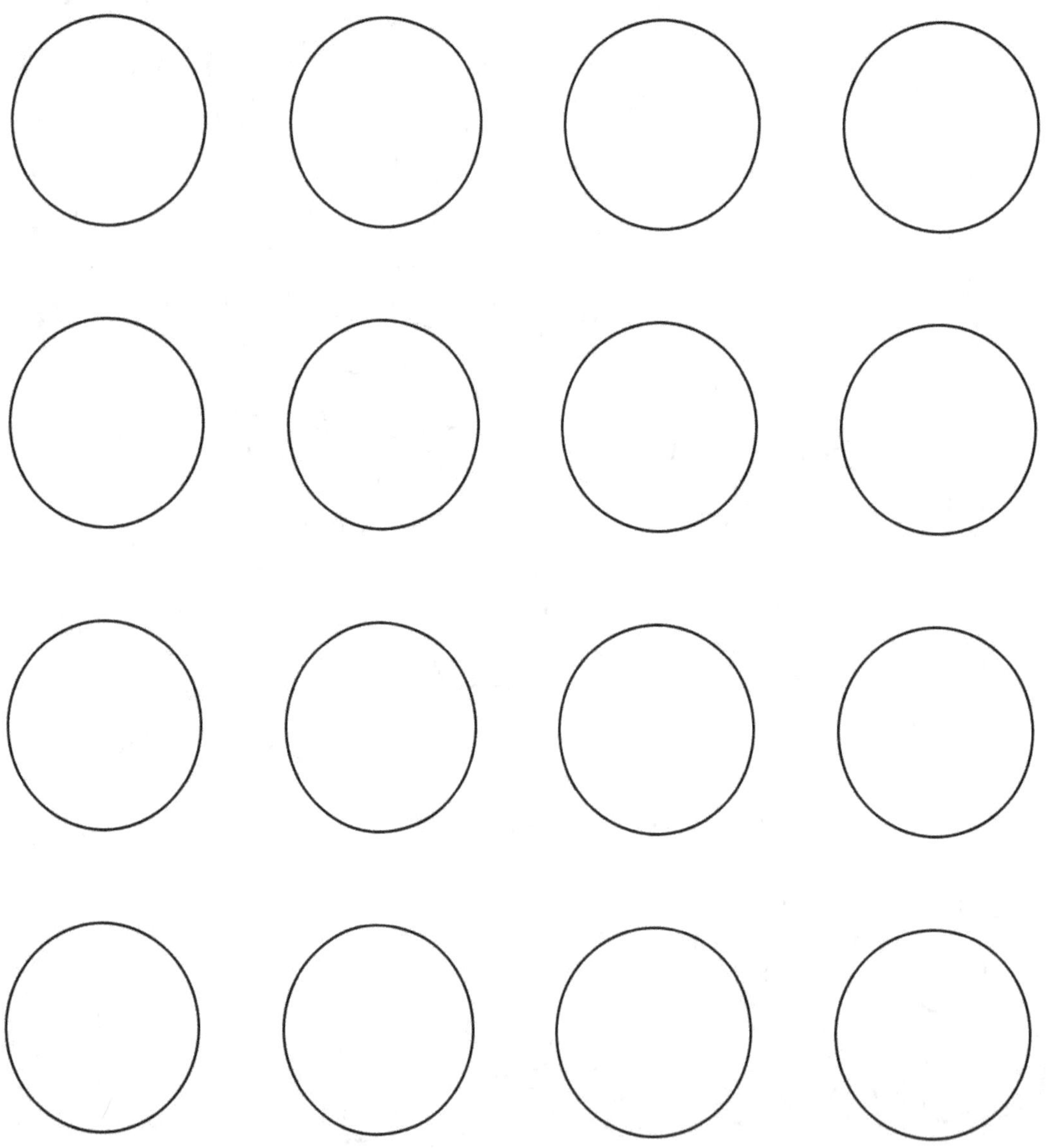

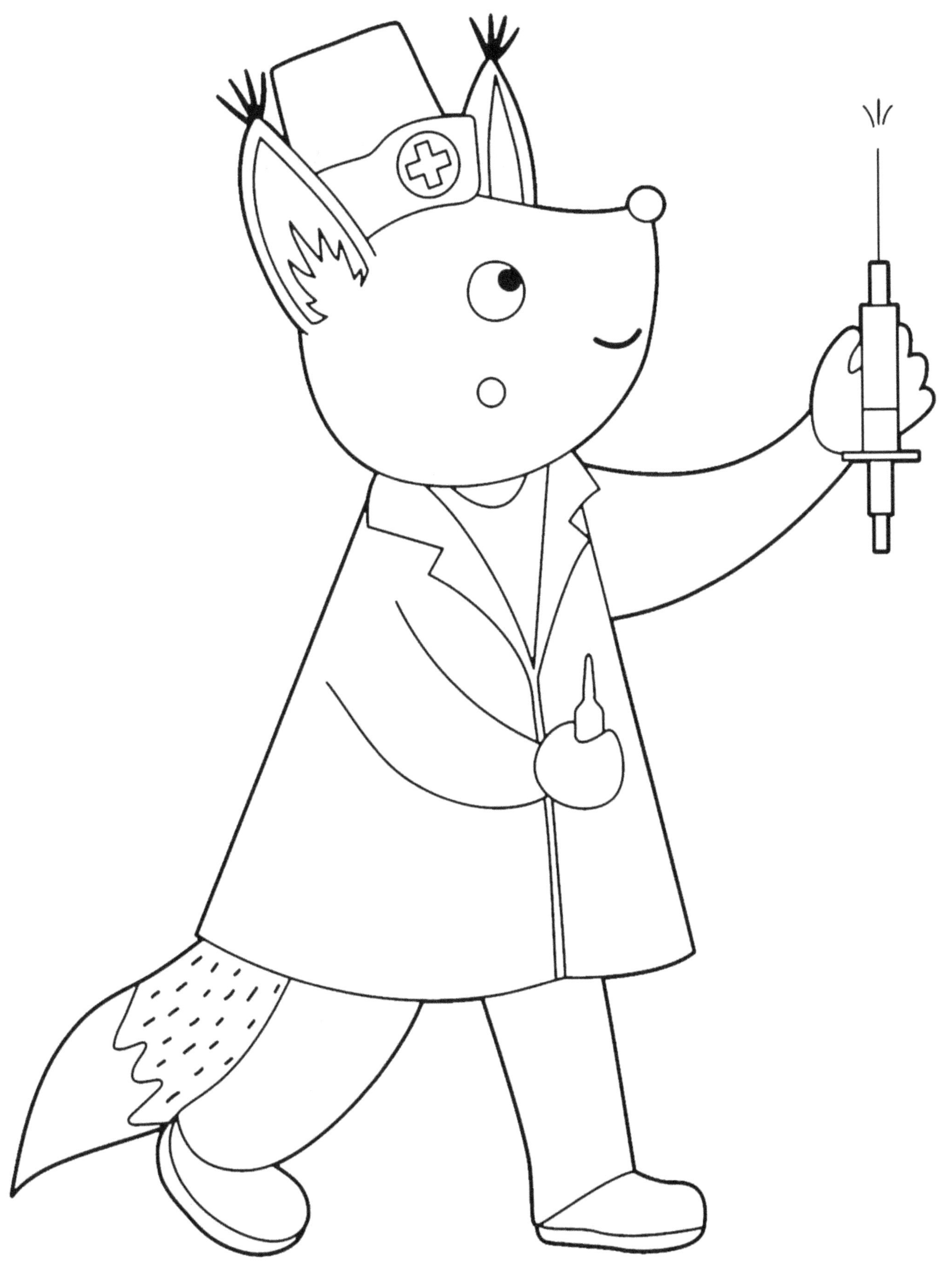

Test Your Color

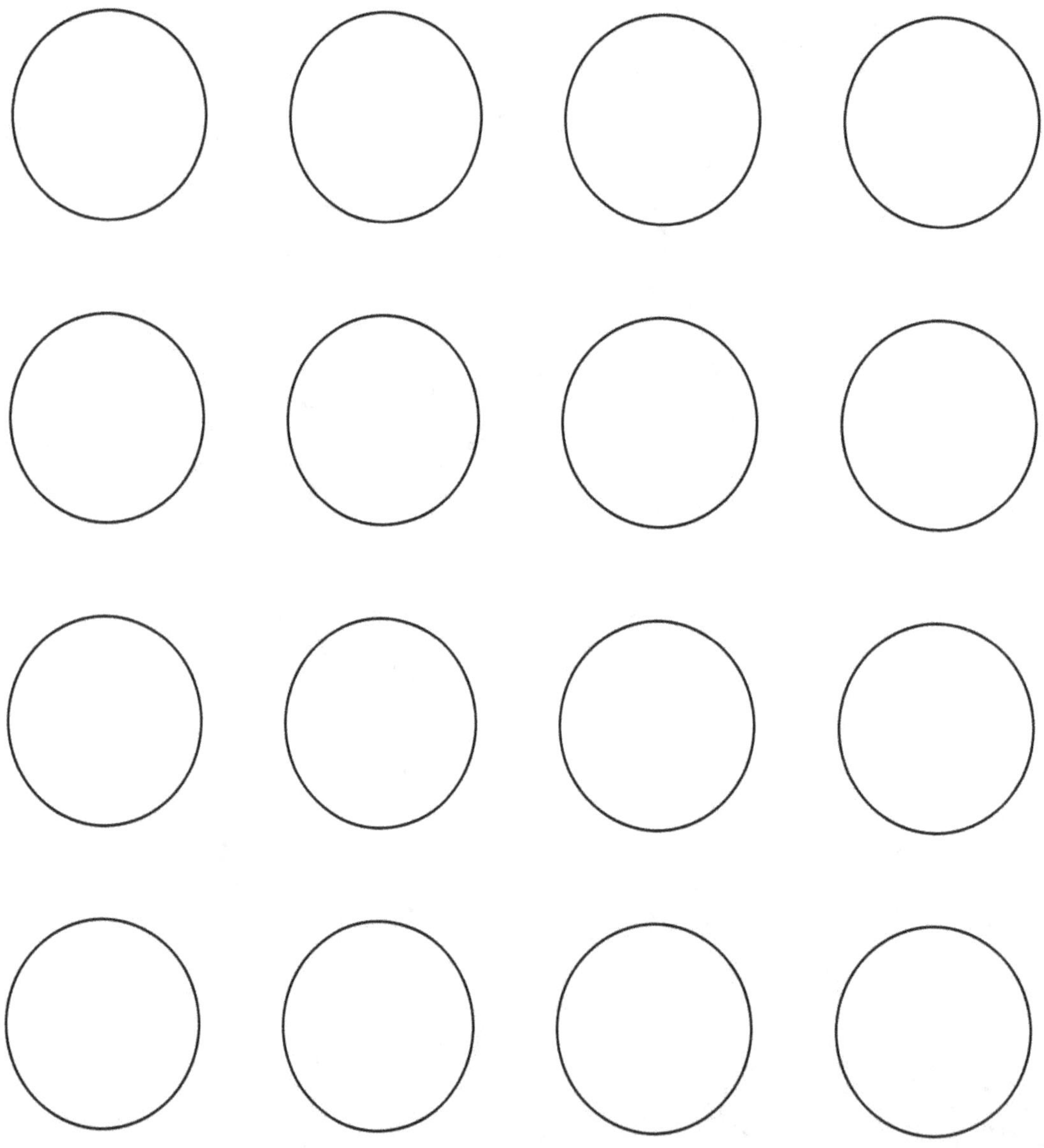

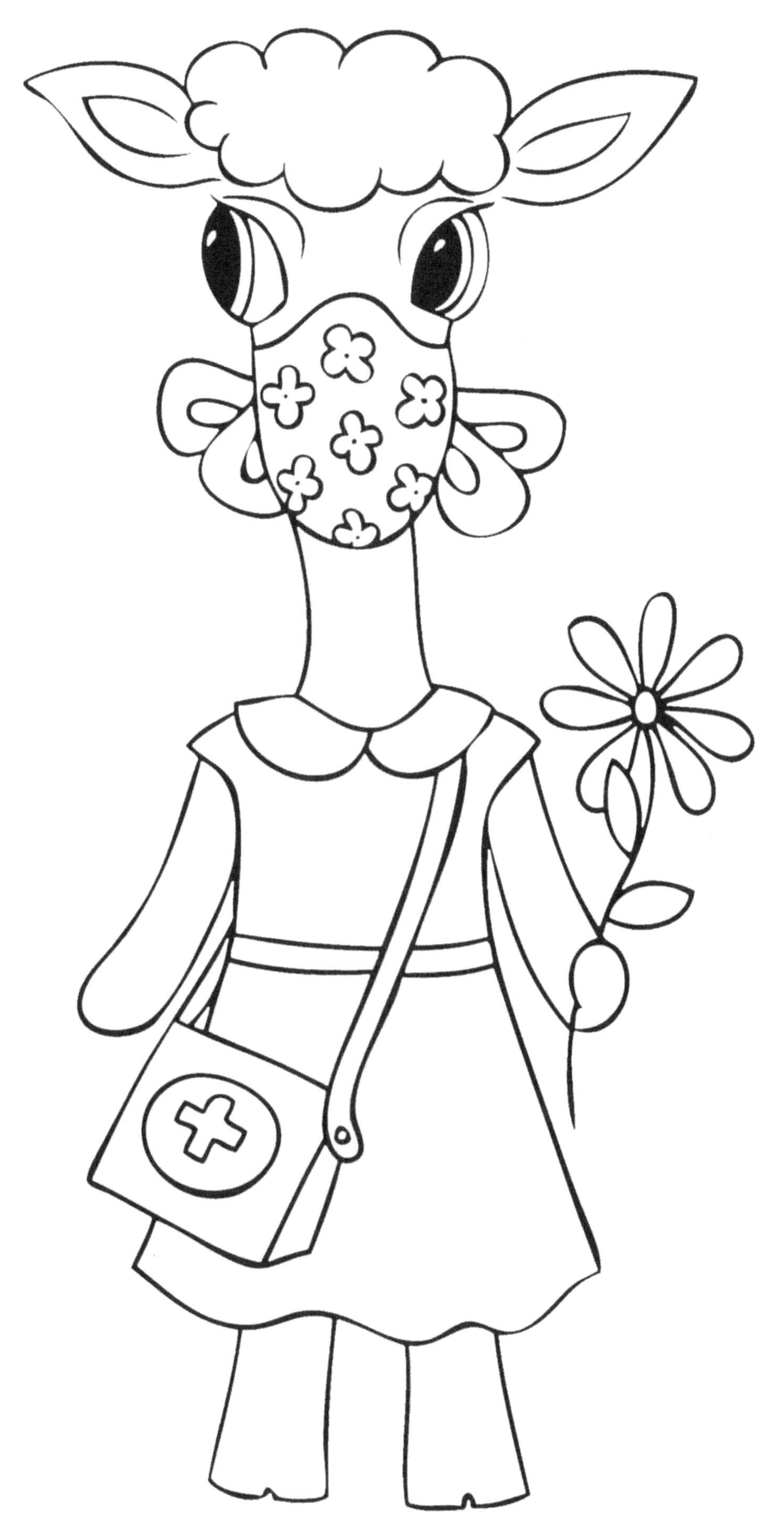

Test Your Color

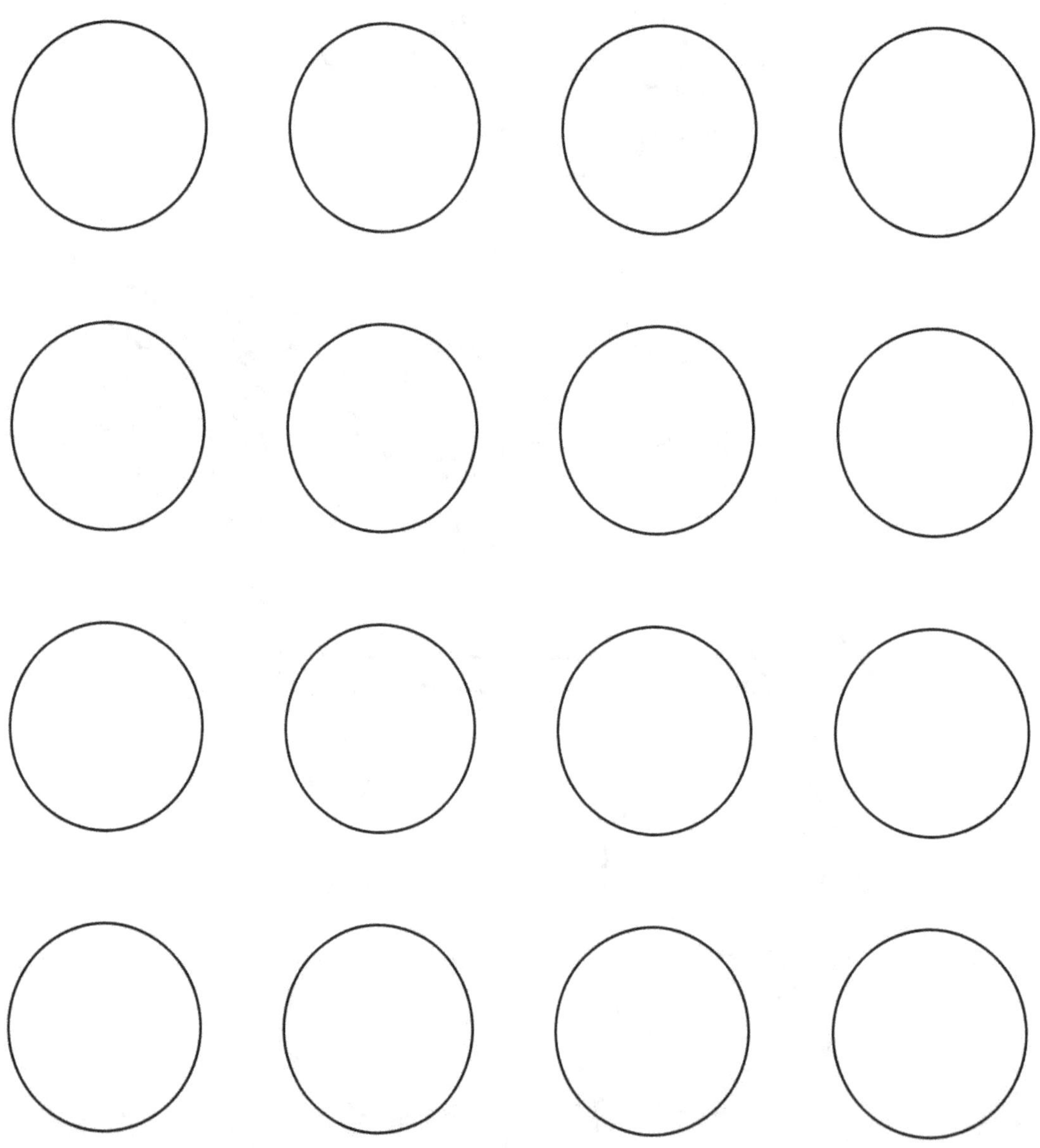

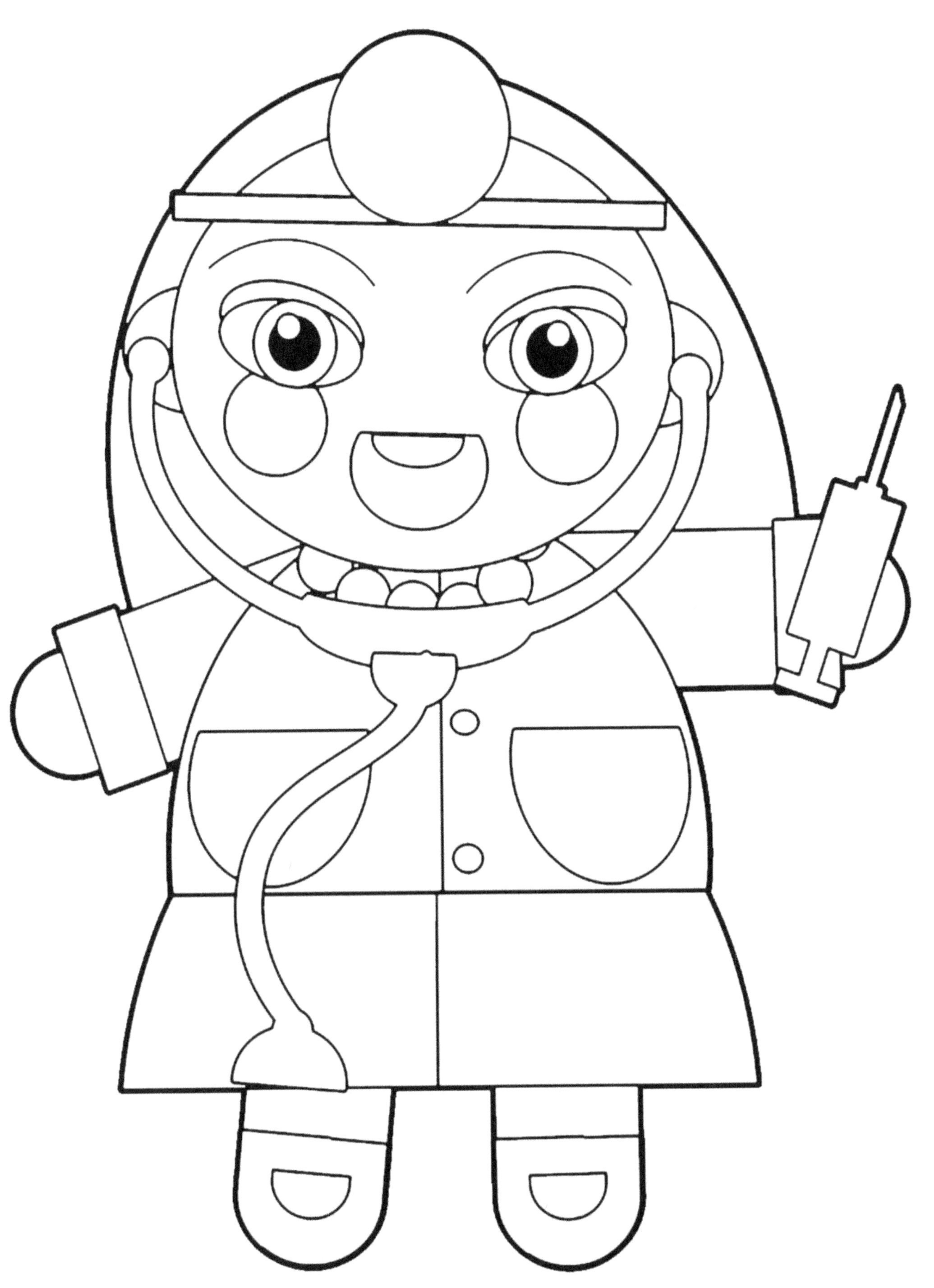

Test Your Color

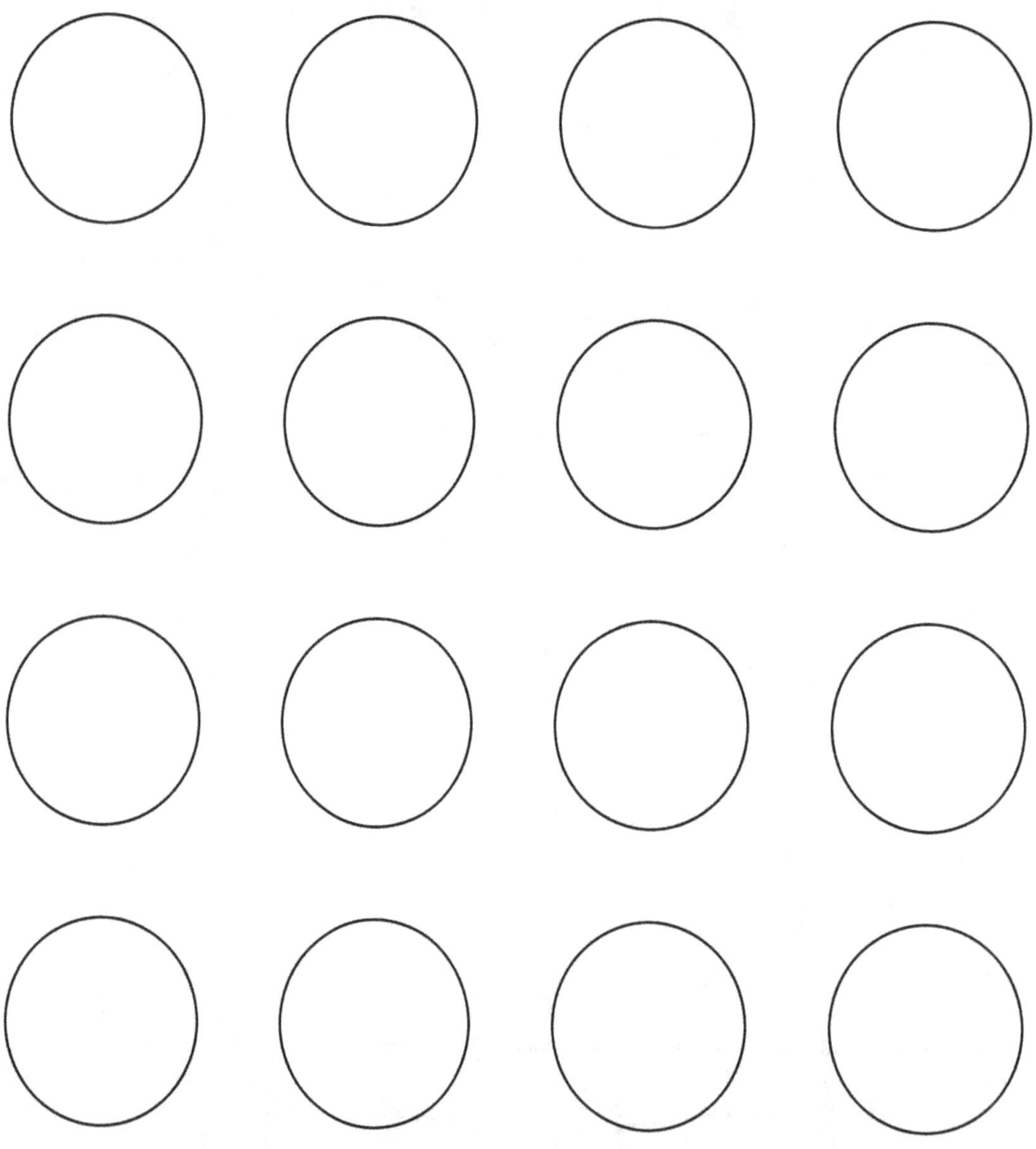

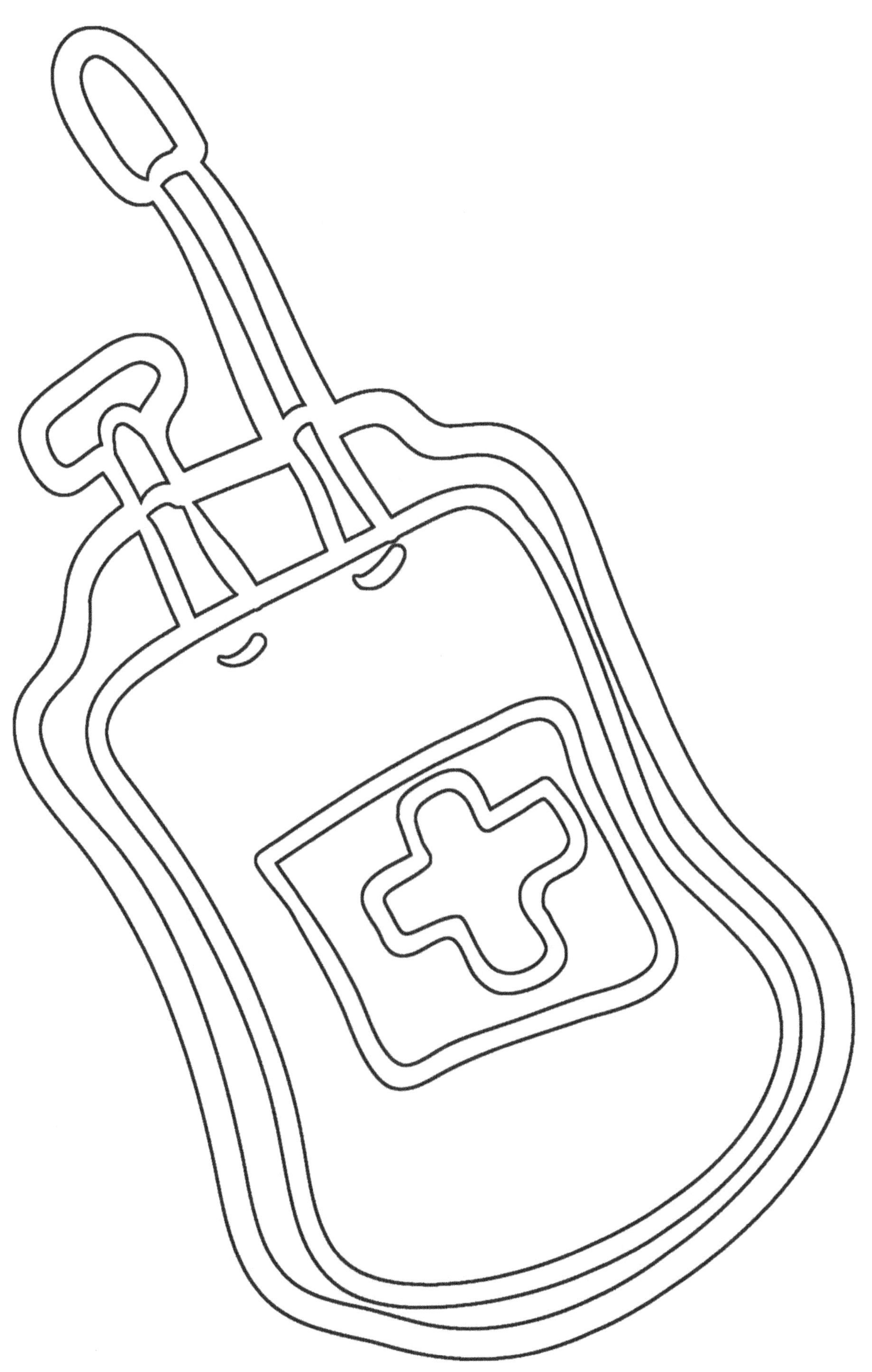

Test Your Color

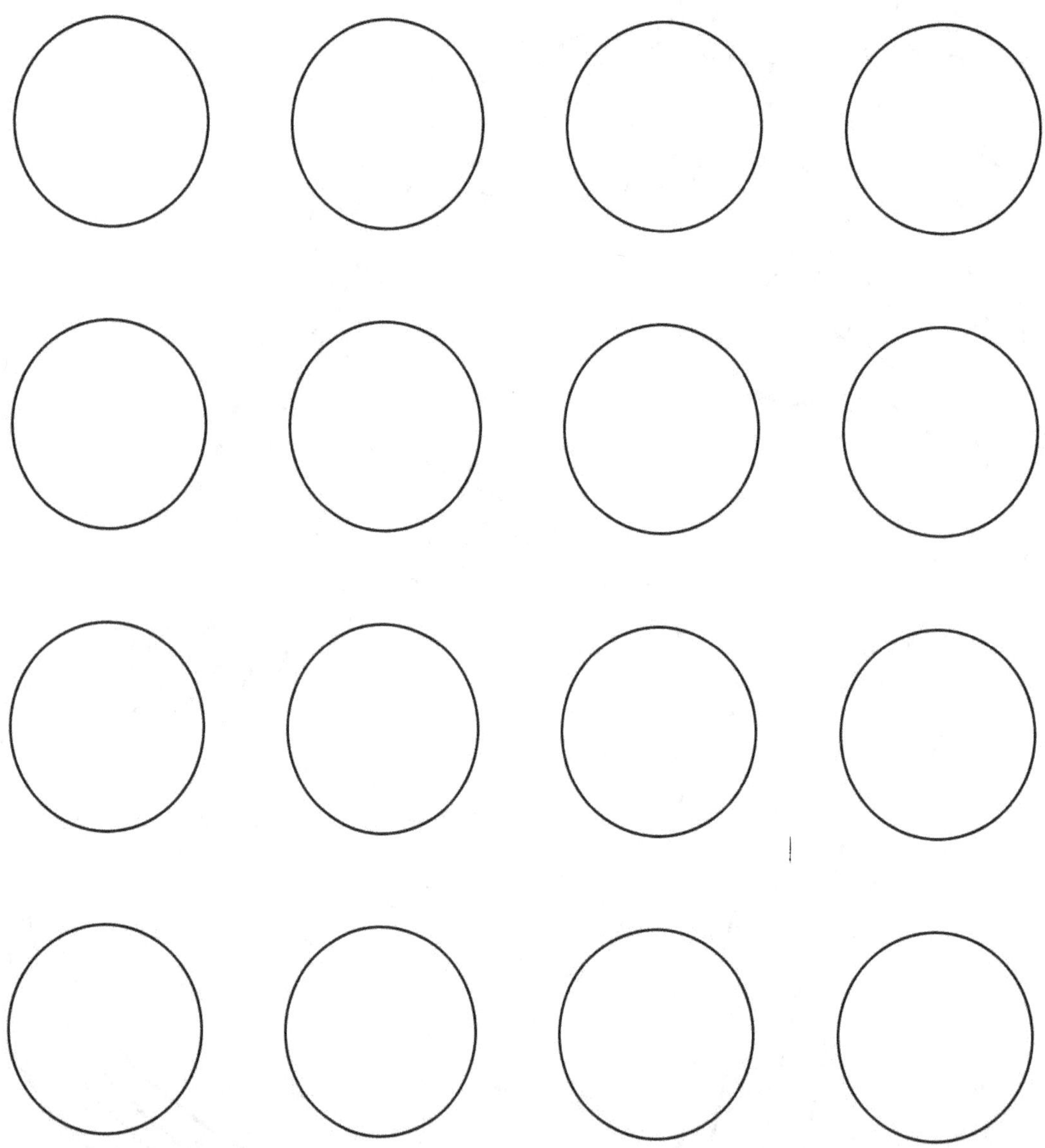

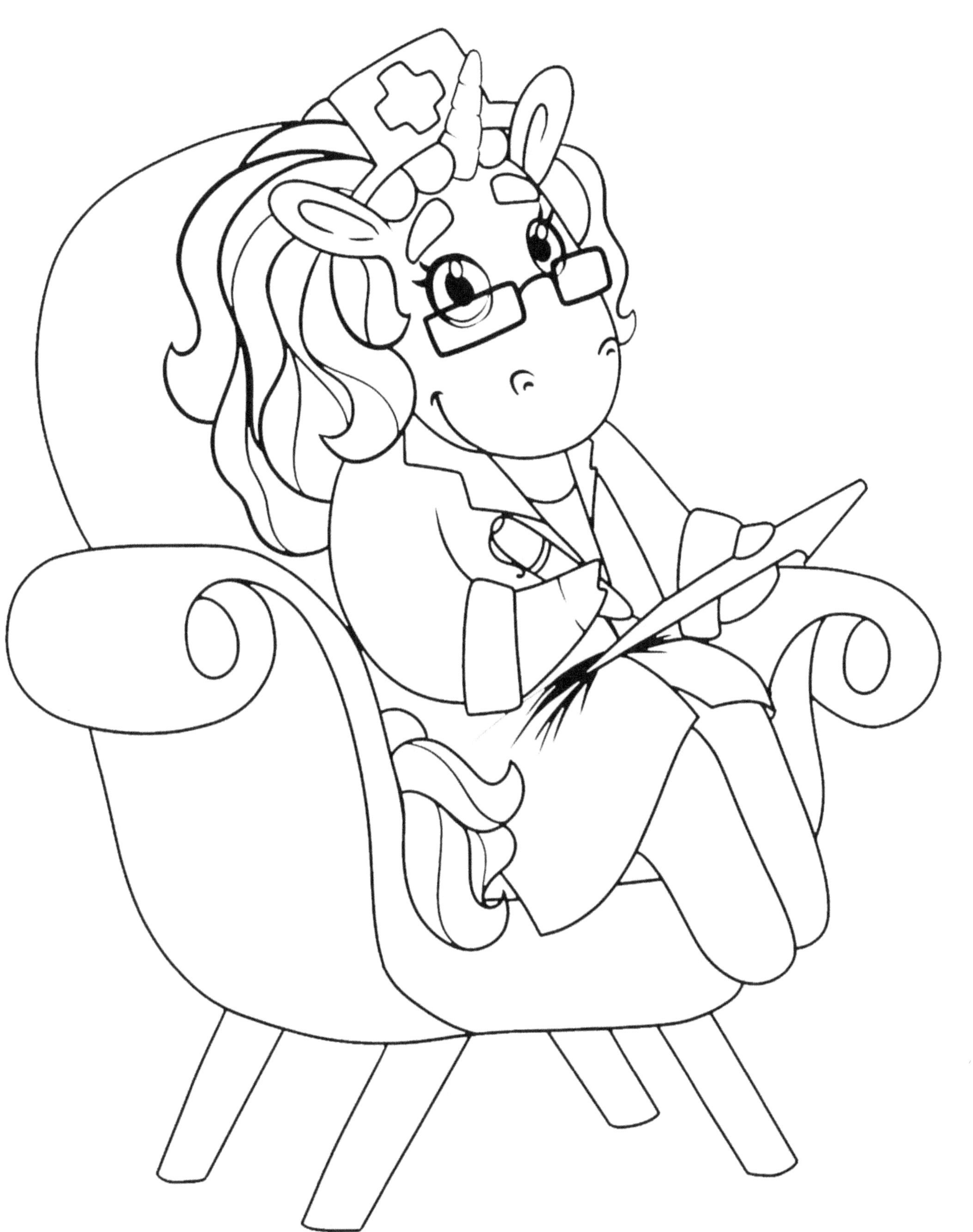

Test Your Color

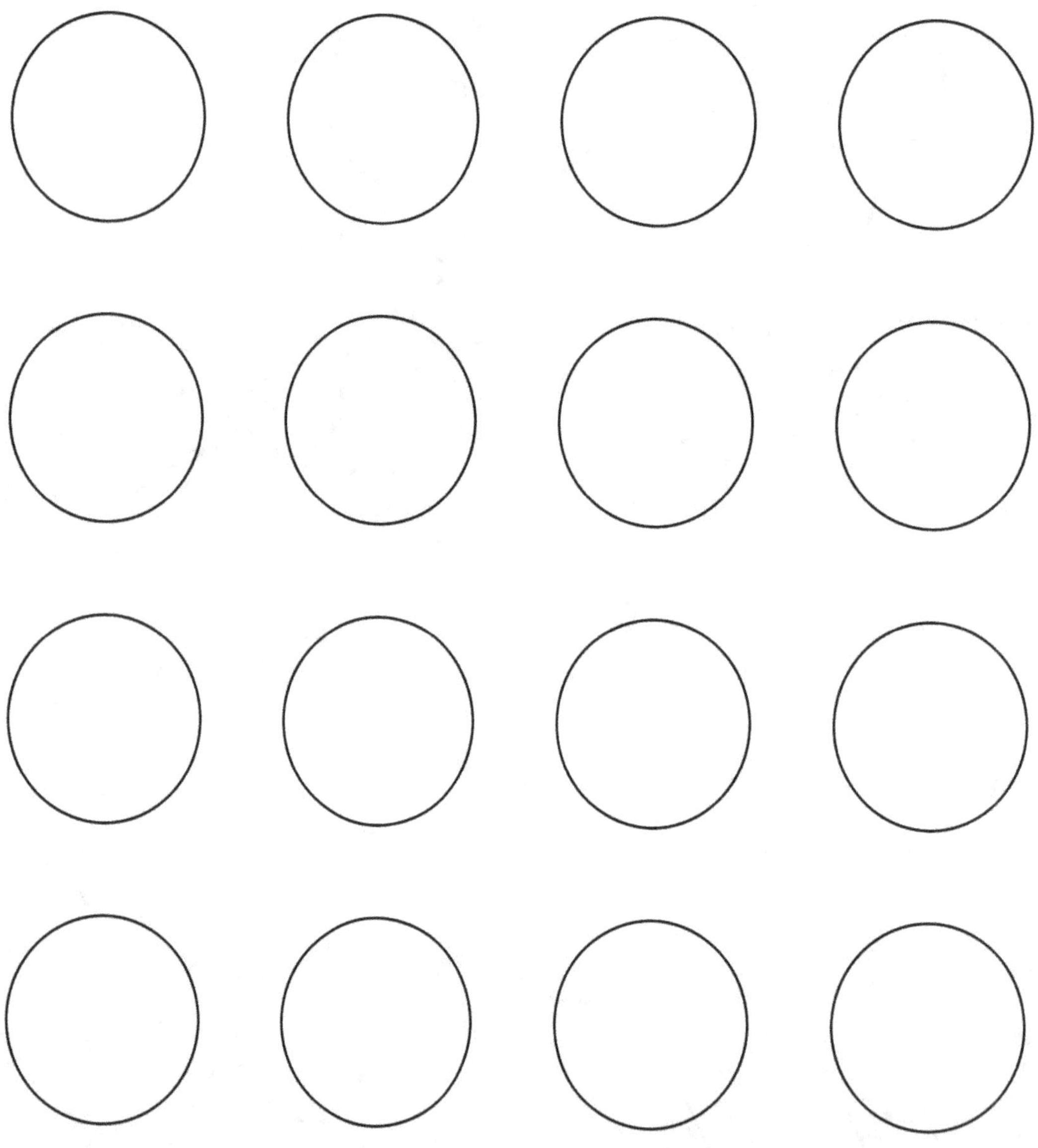

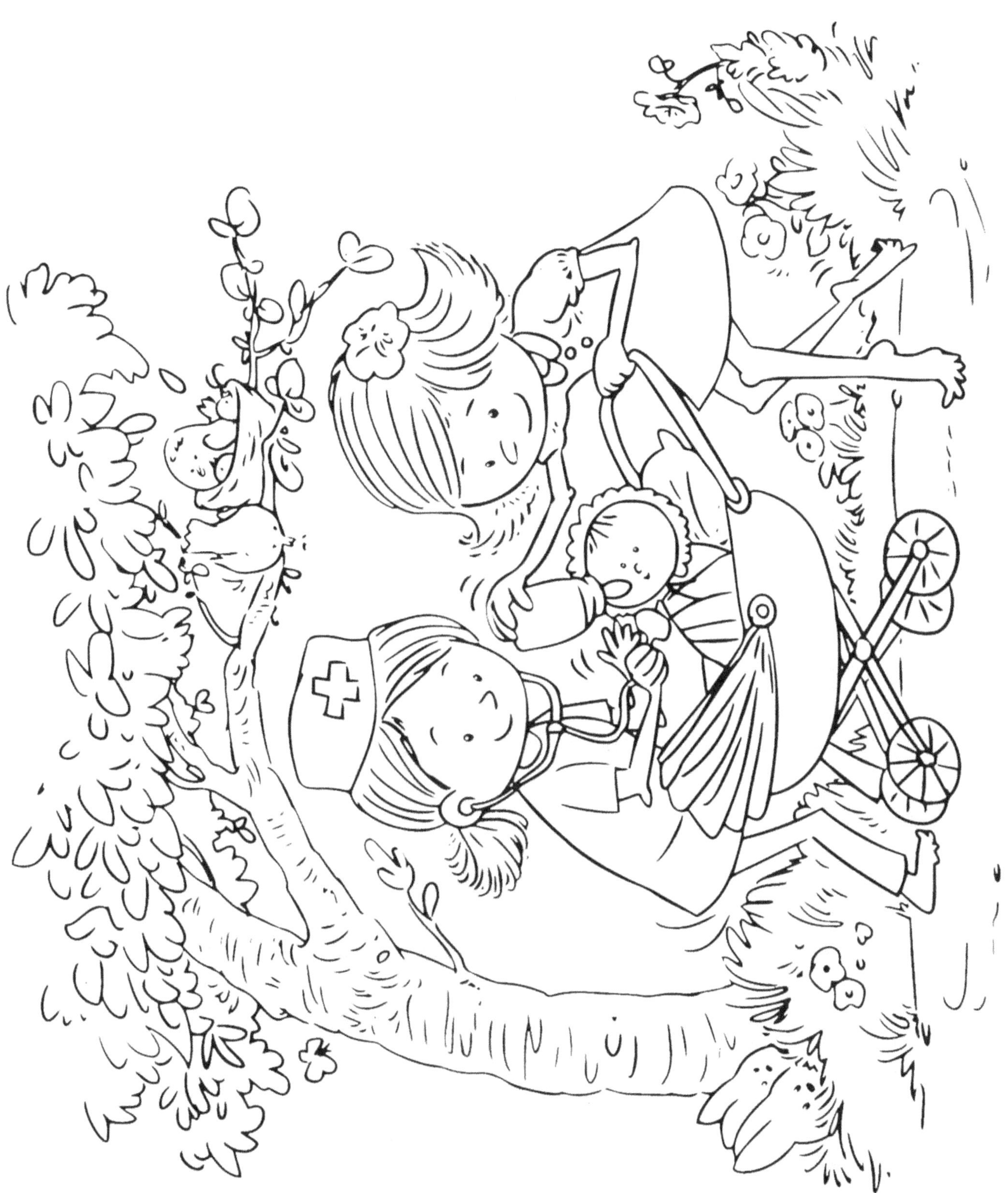

Test Your Color

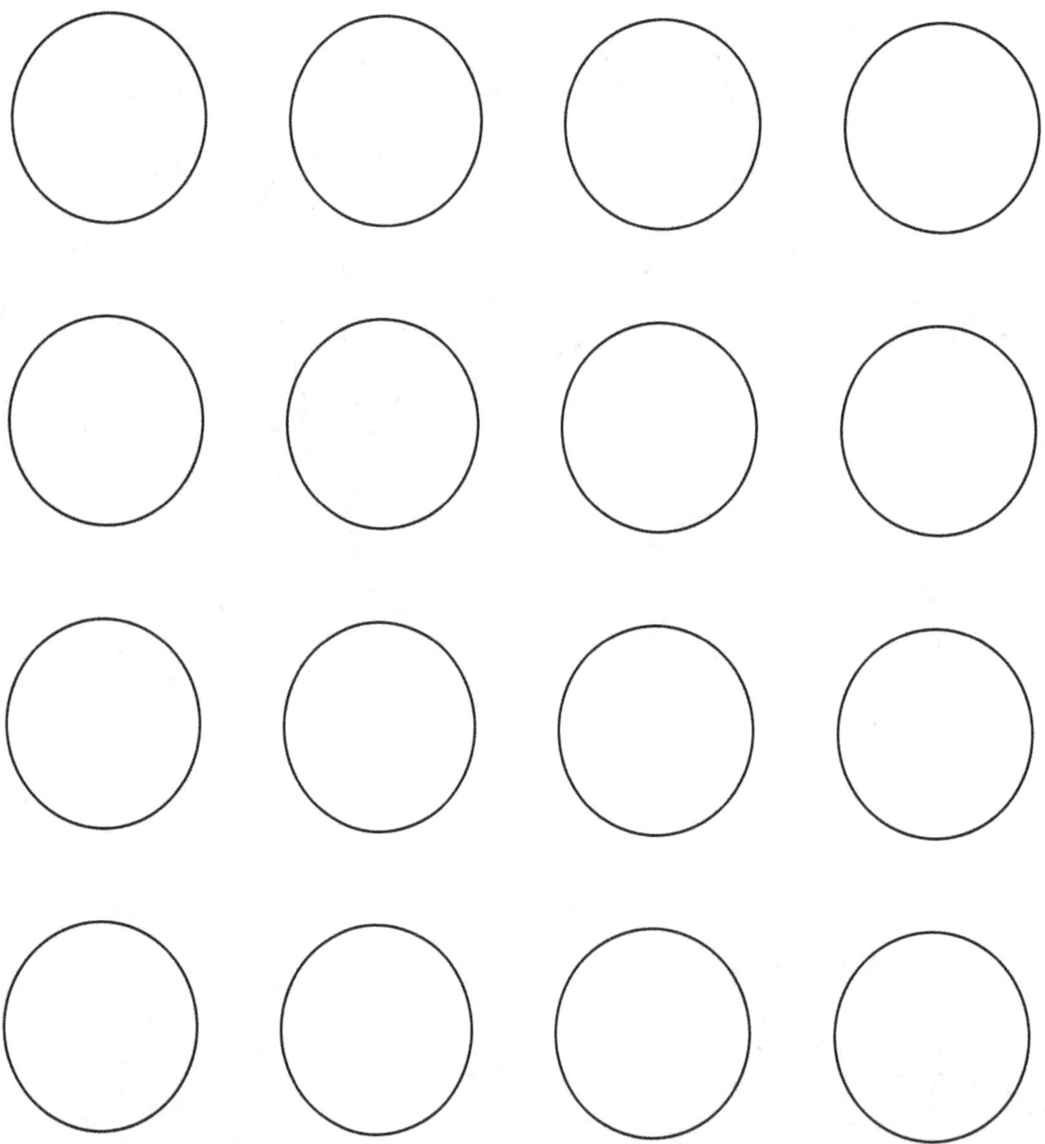

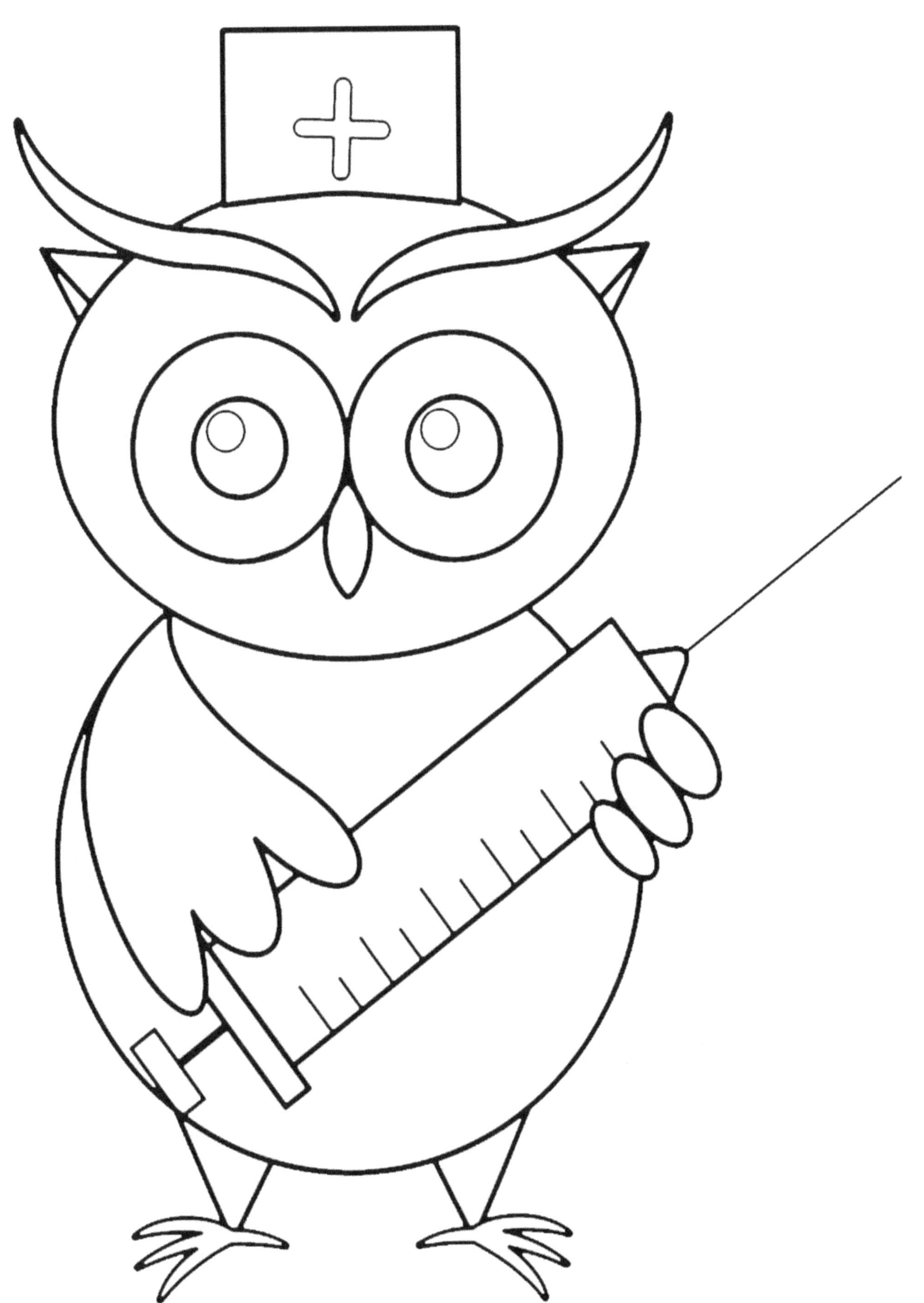

Test Your Color

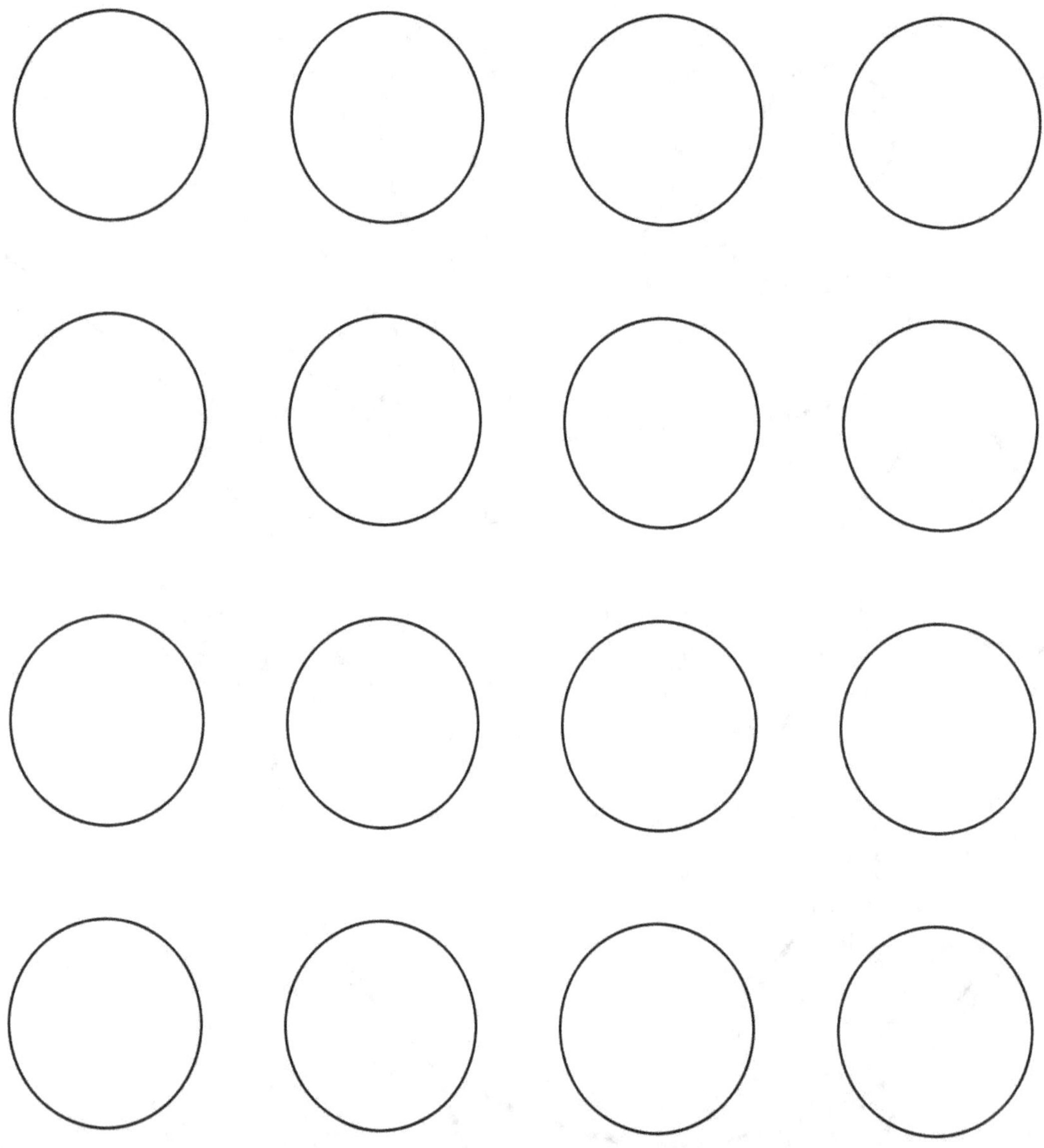

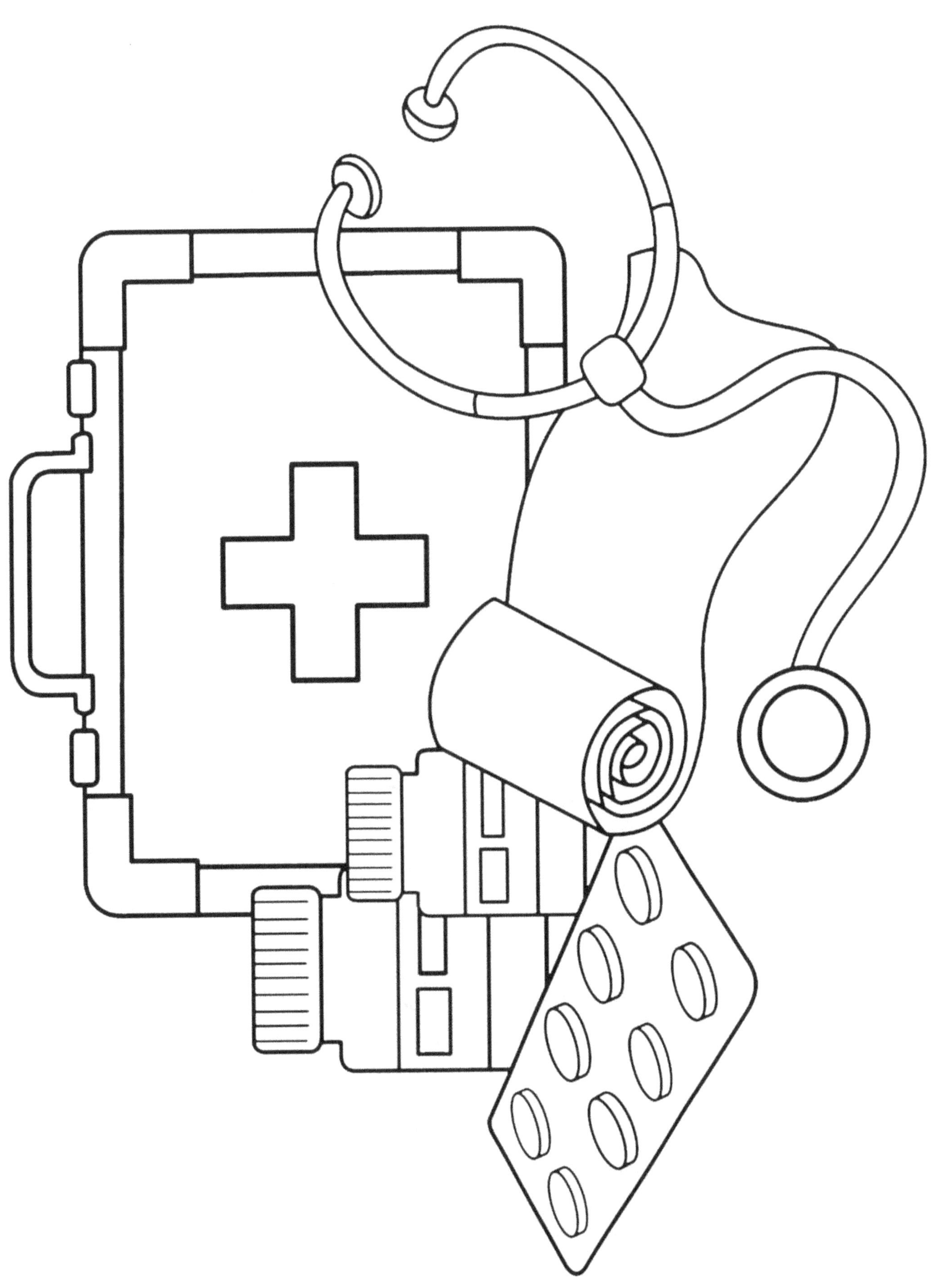

Test Your Color

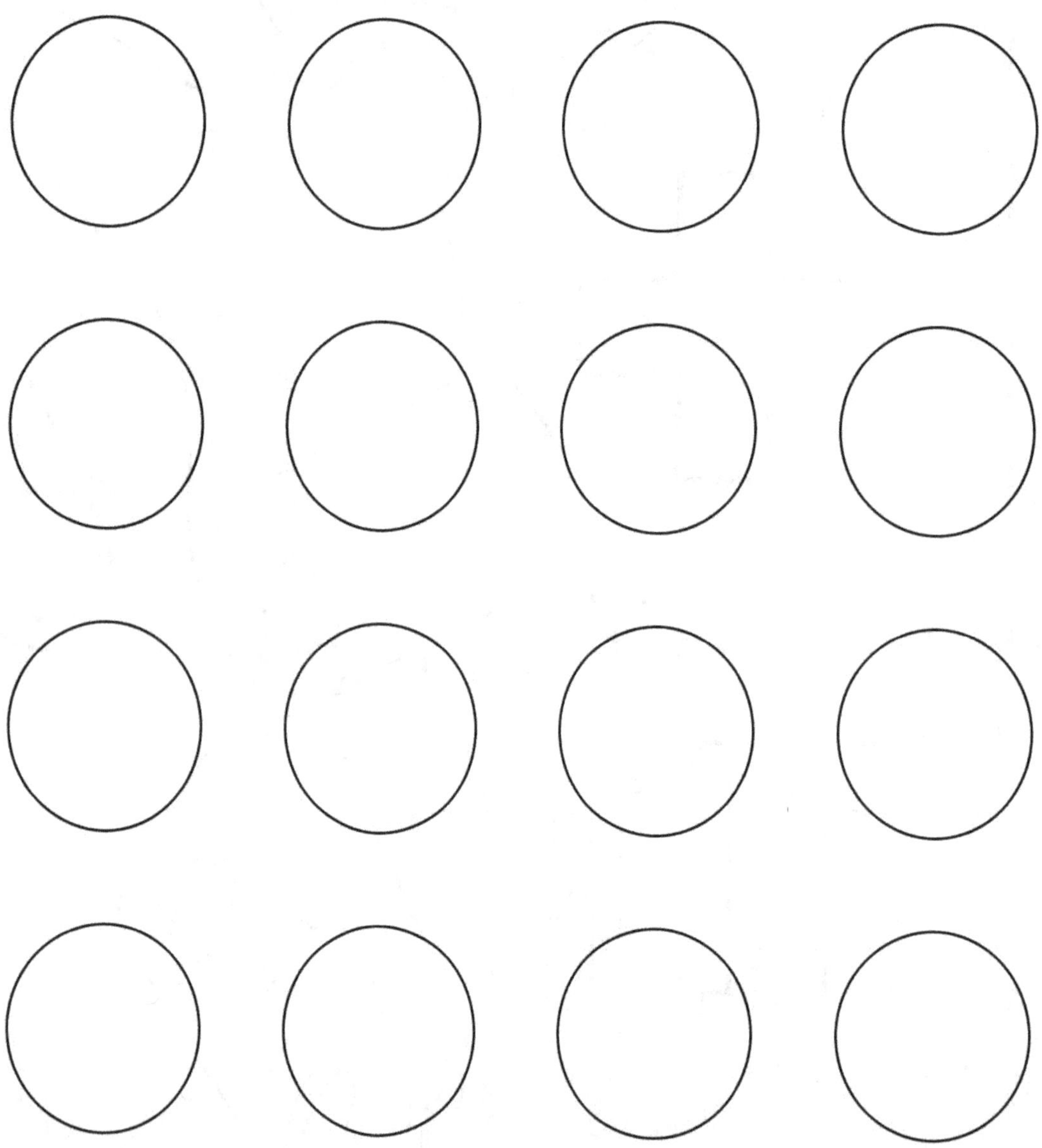

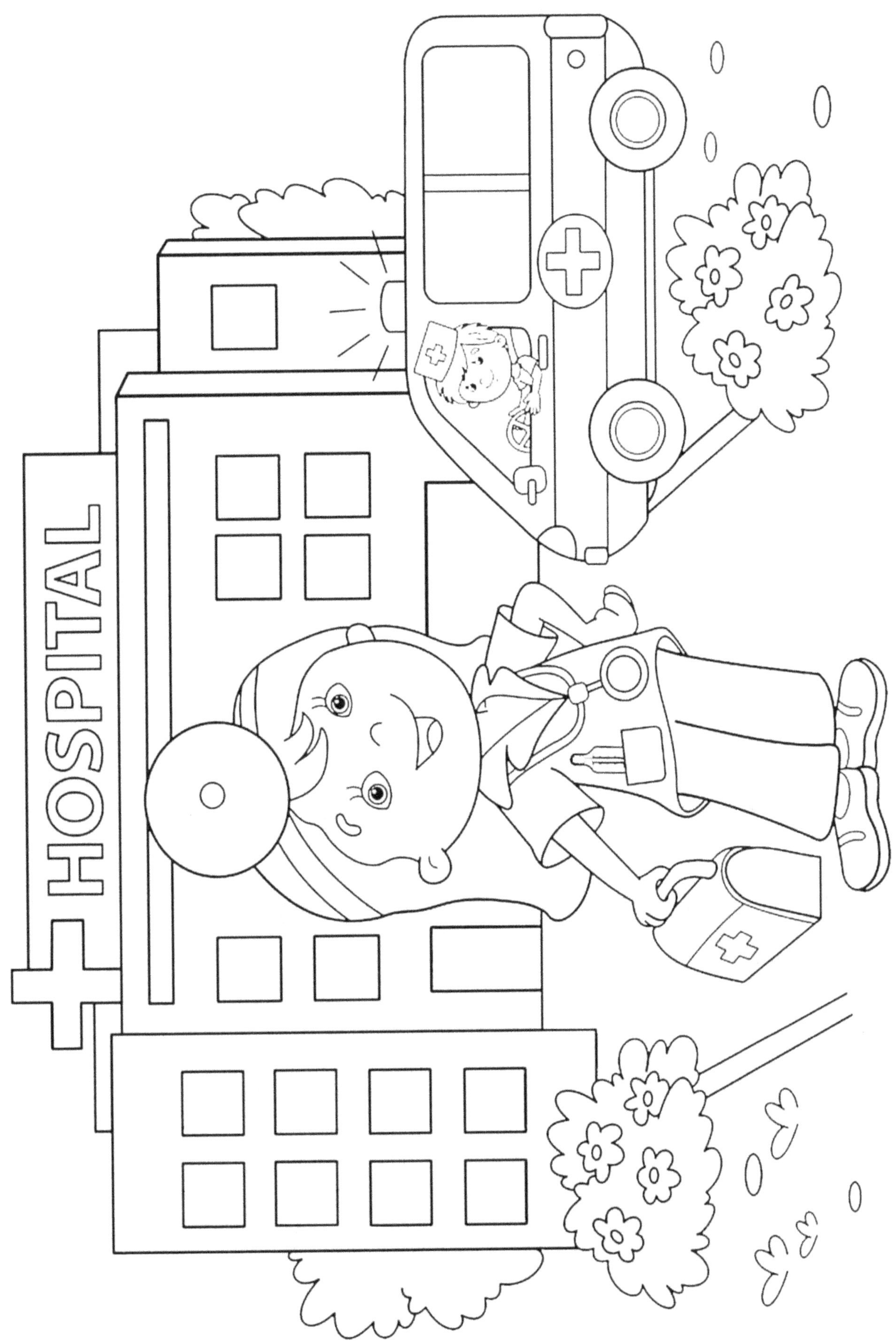

HOSPITAL

Test Your Color

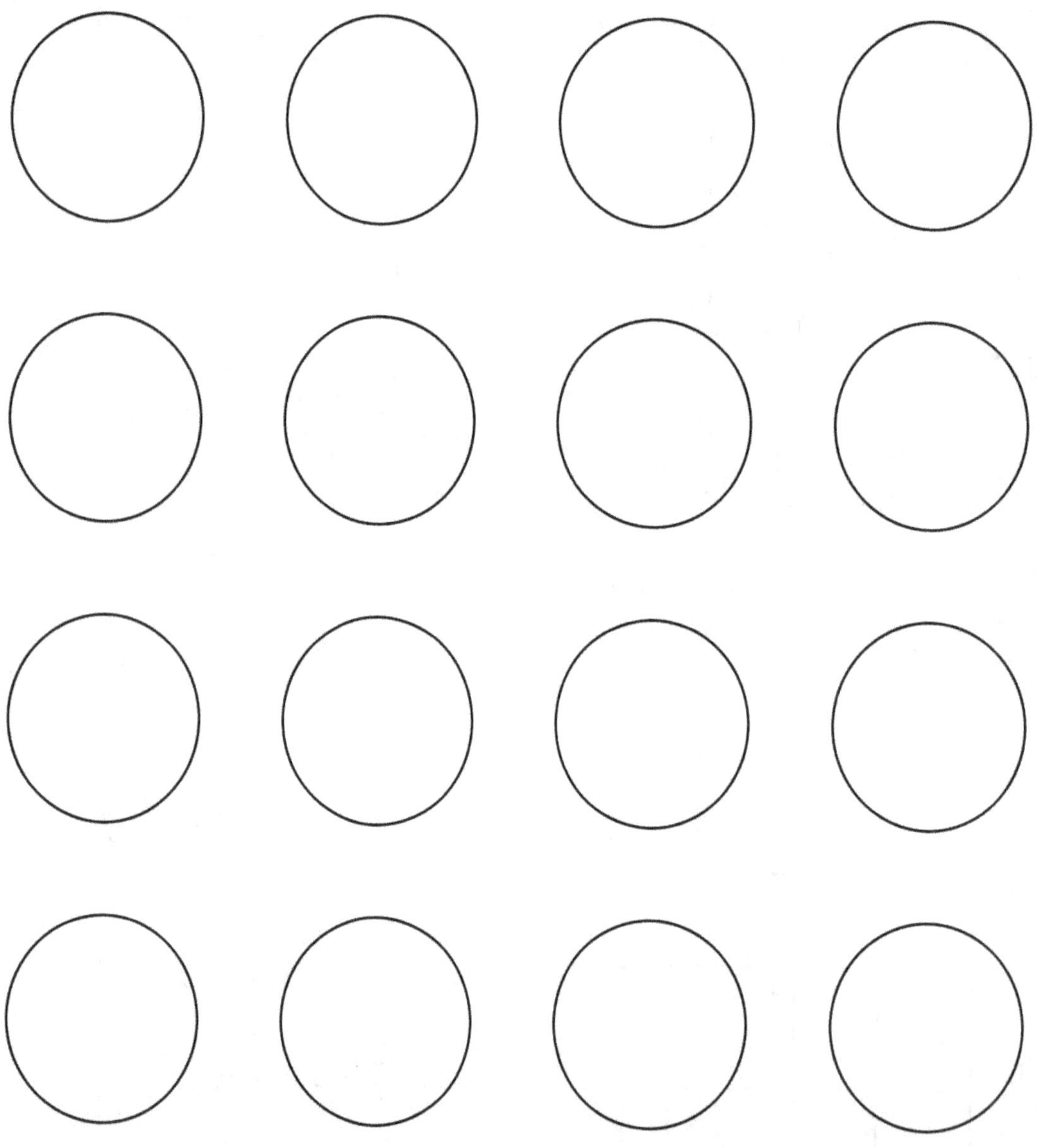

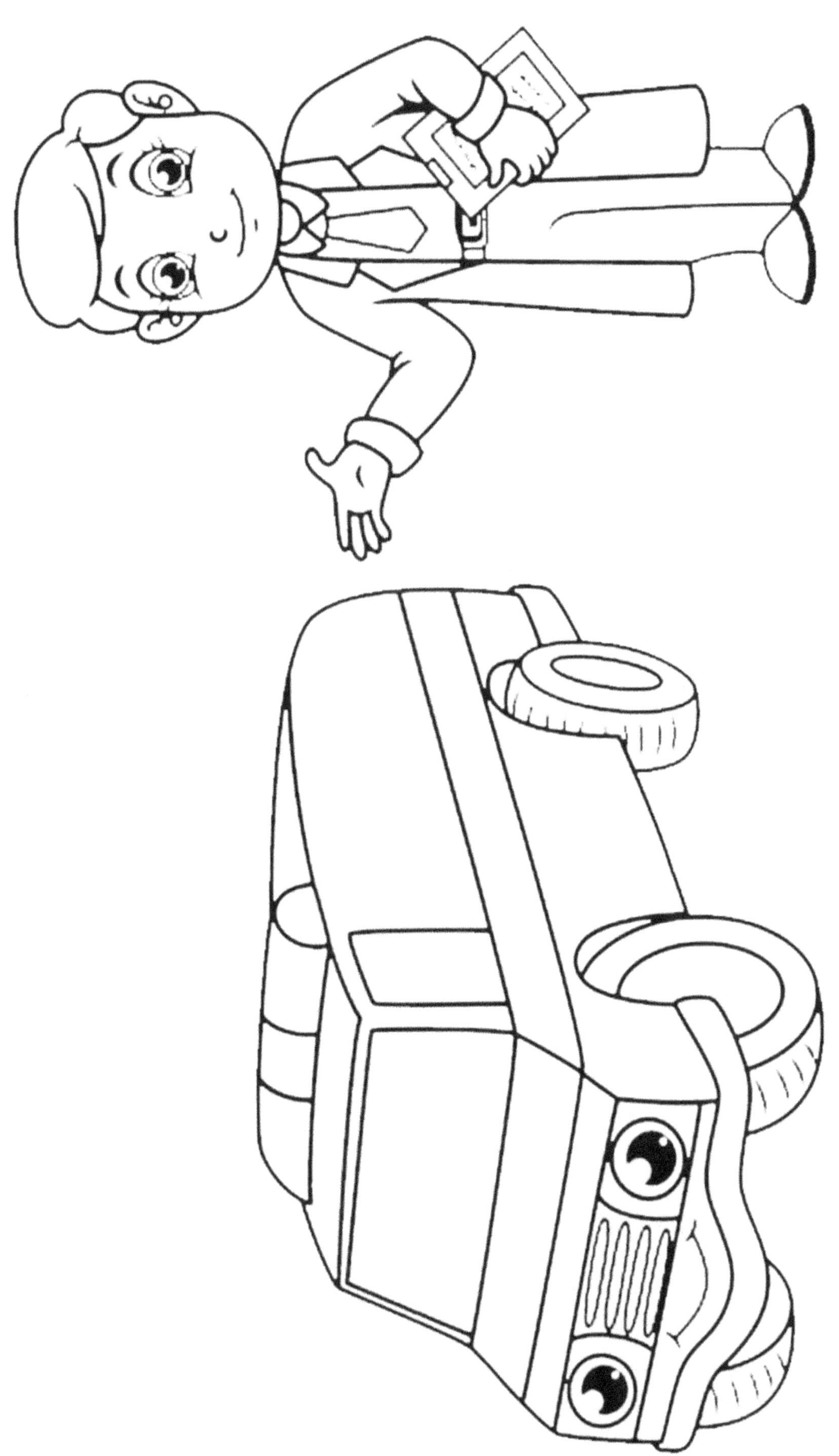

Test Your Color

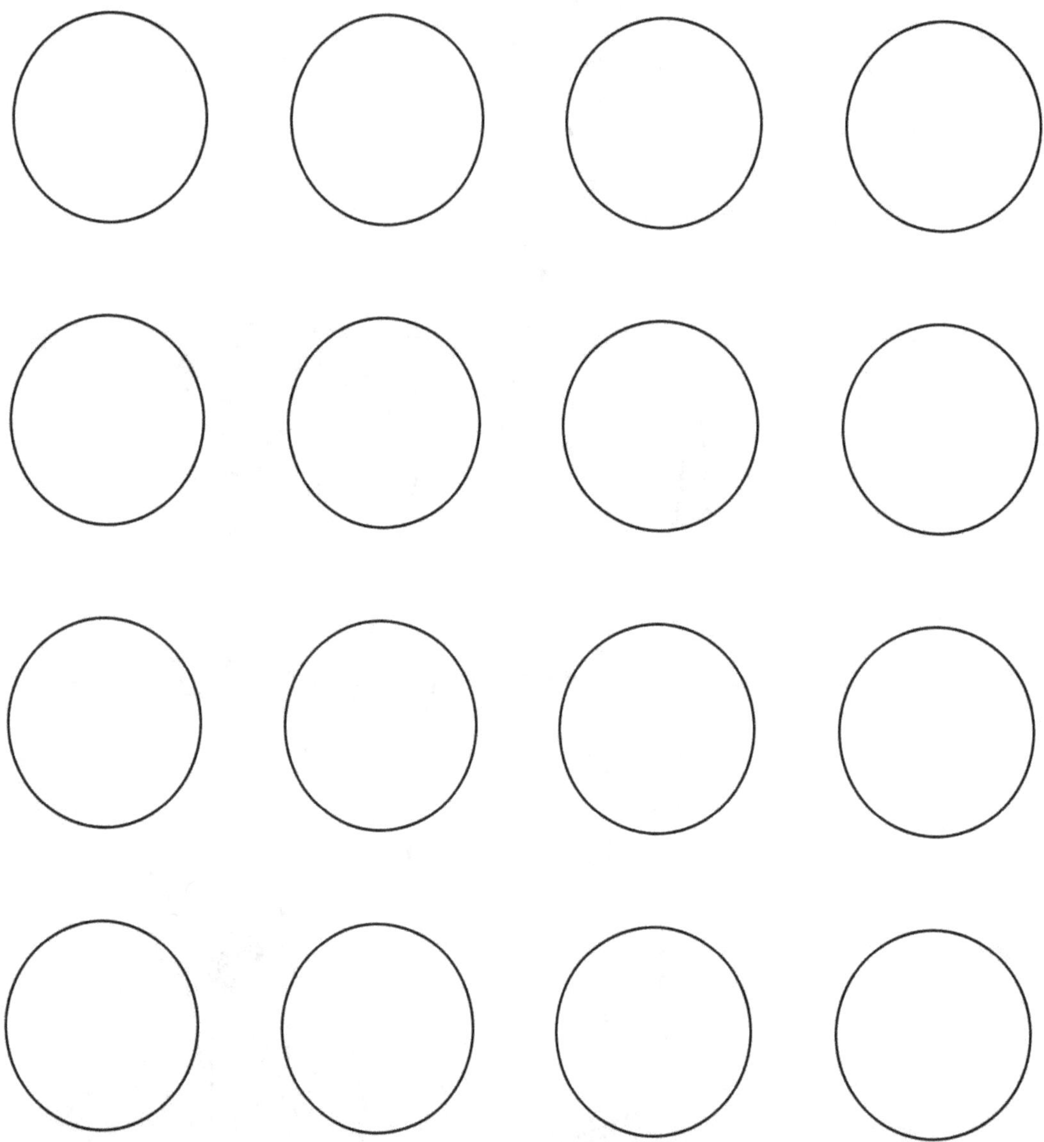

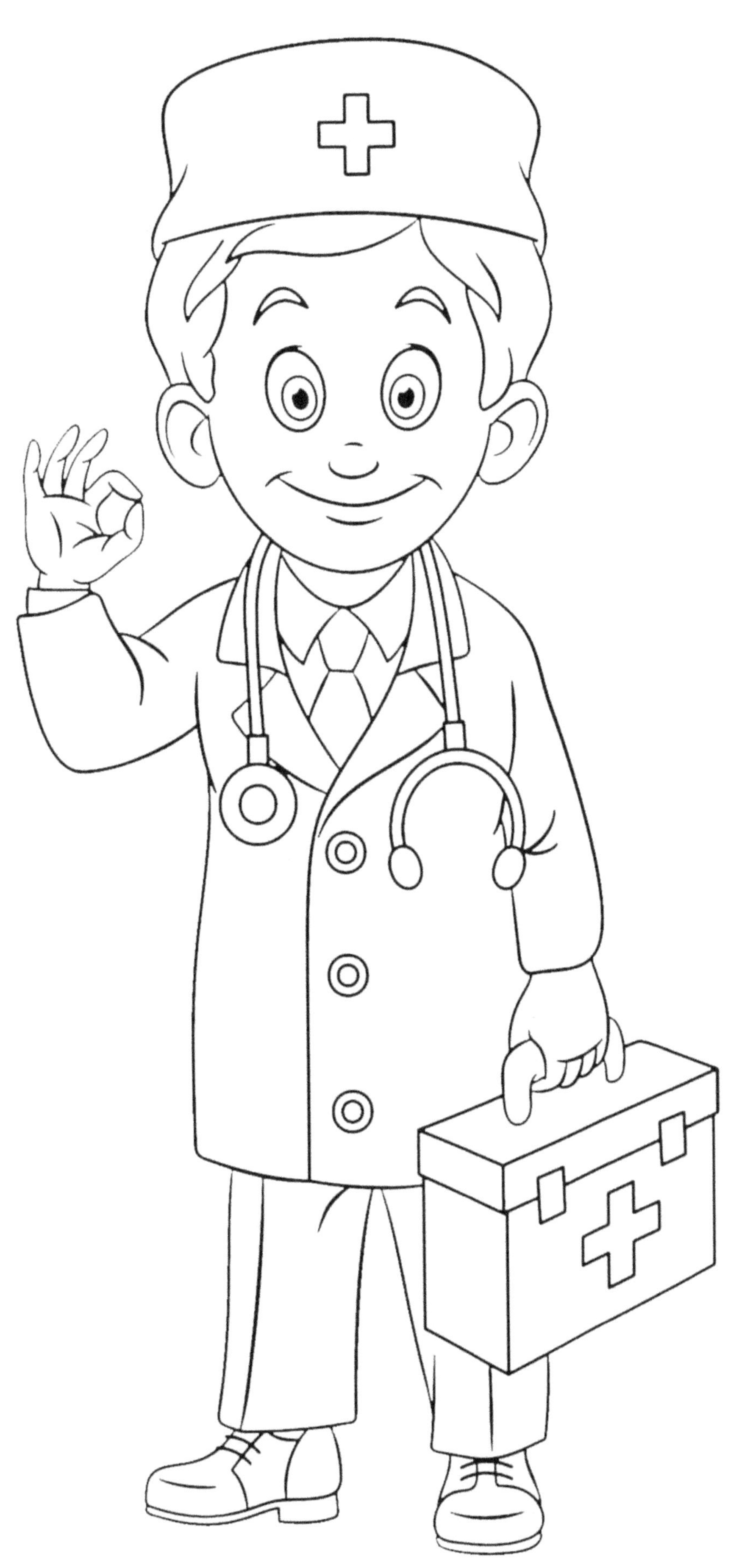

Test Your Color

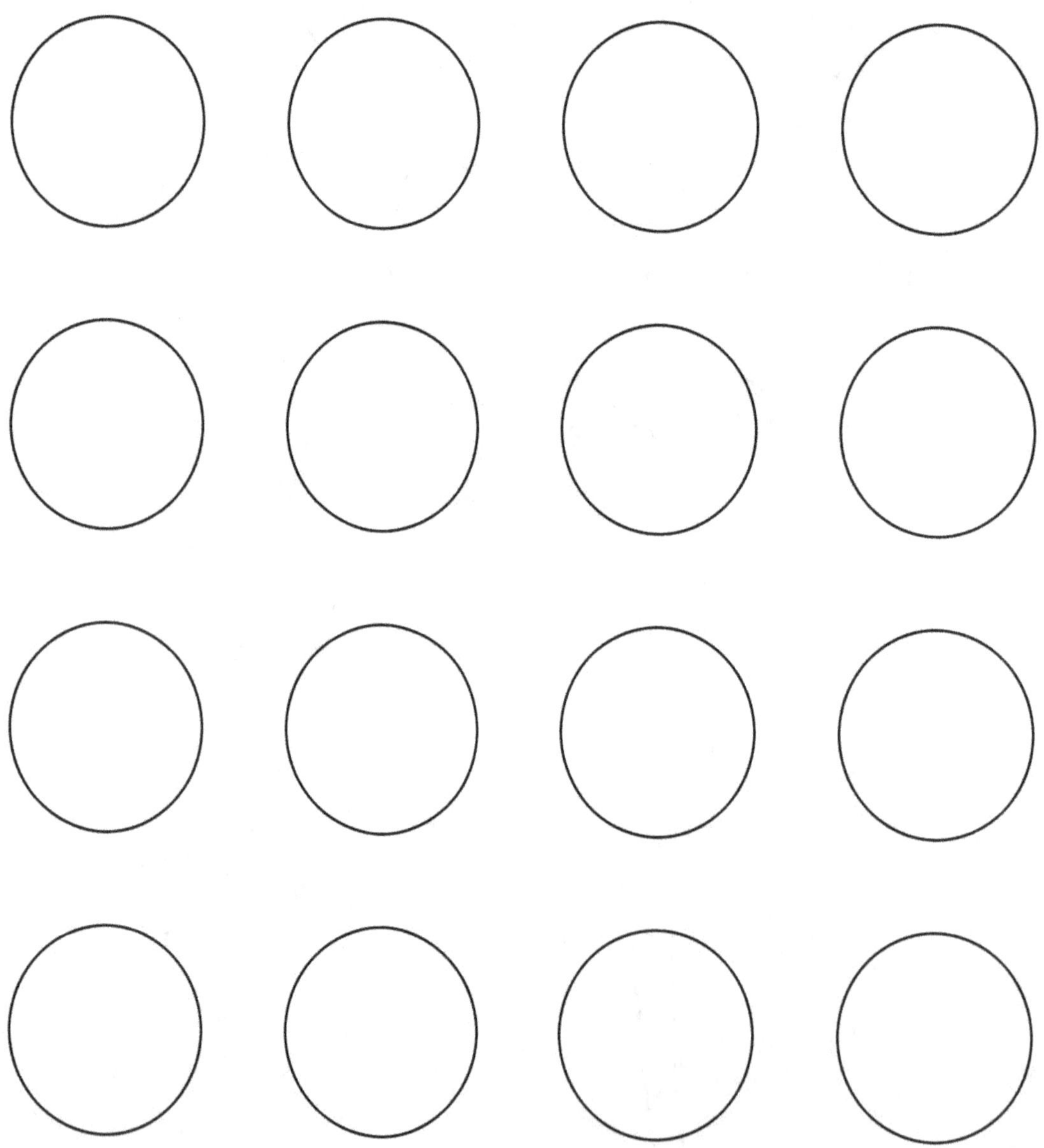

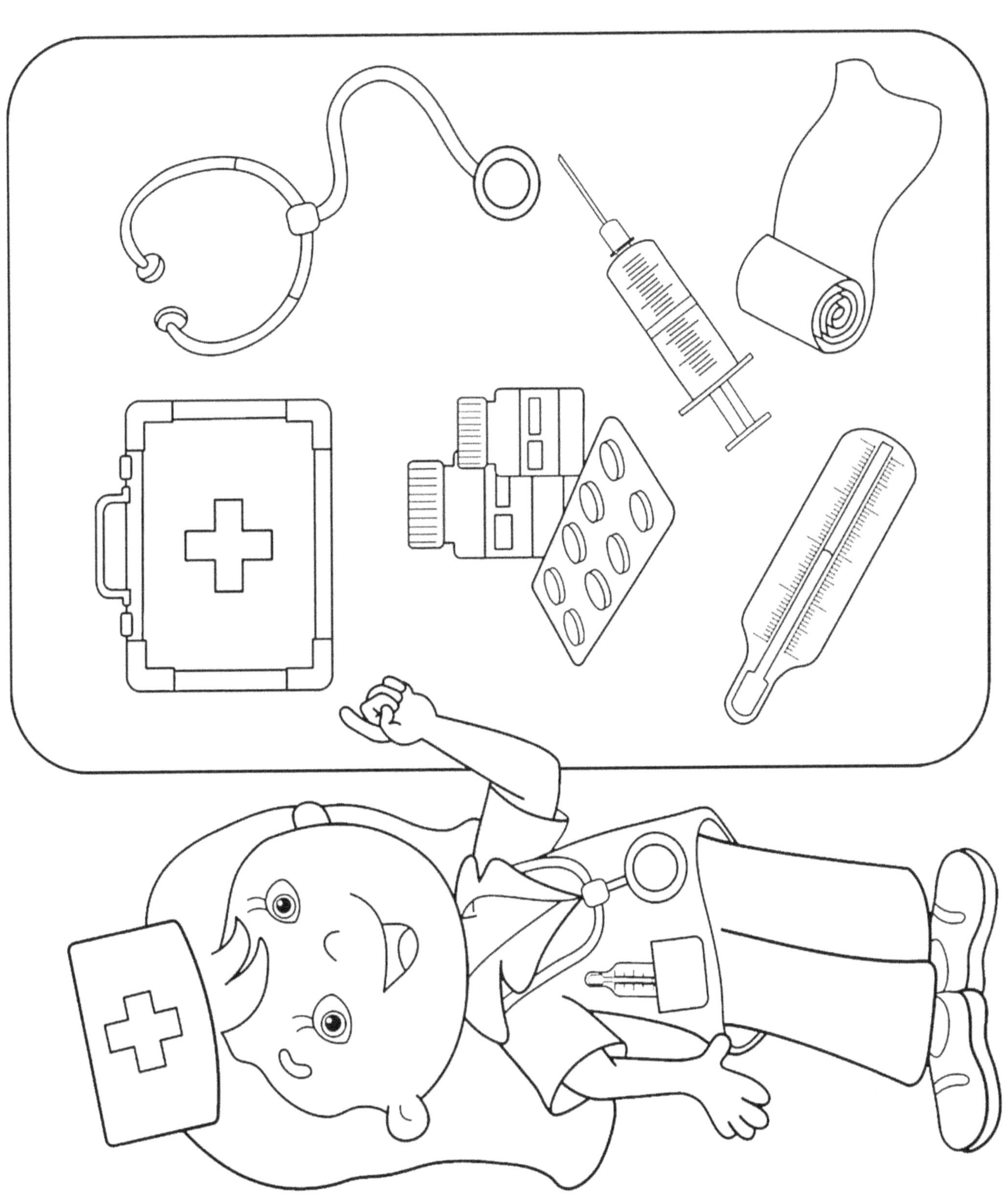

Test Your Color

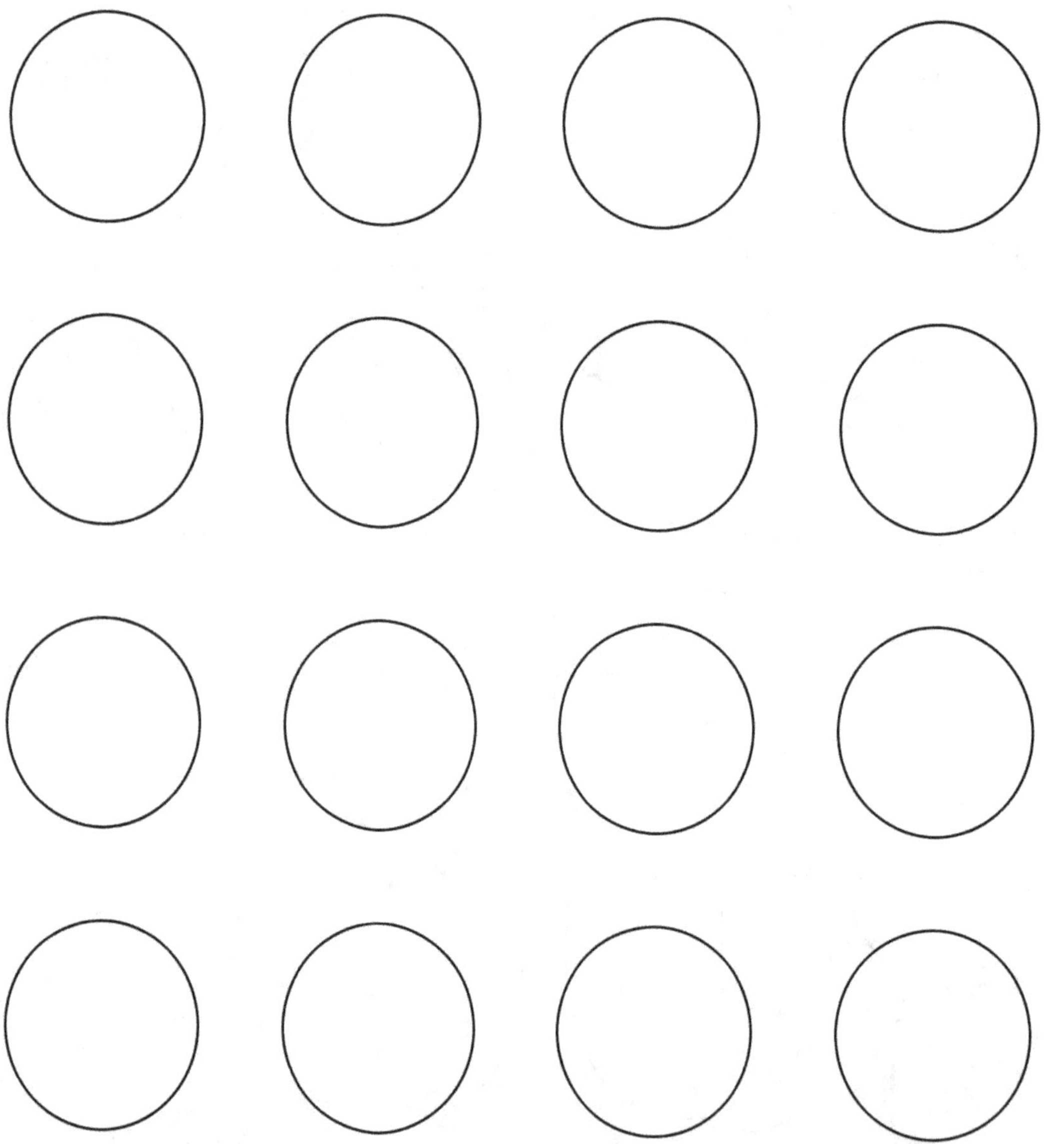

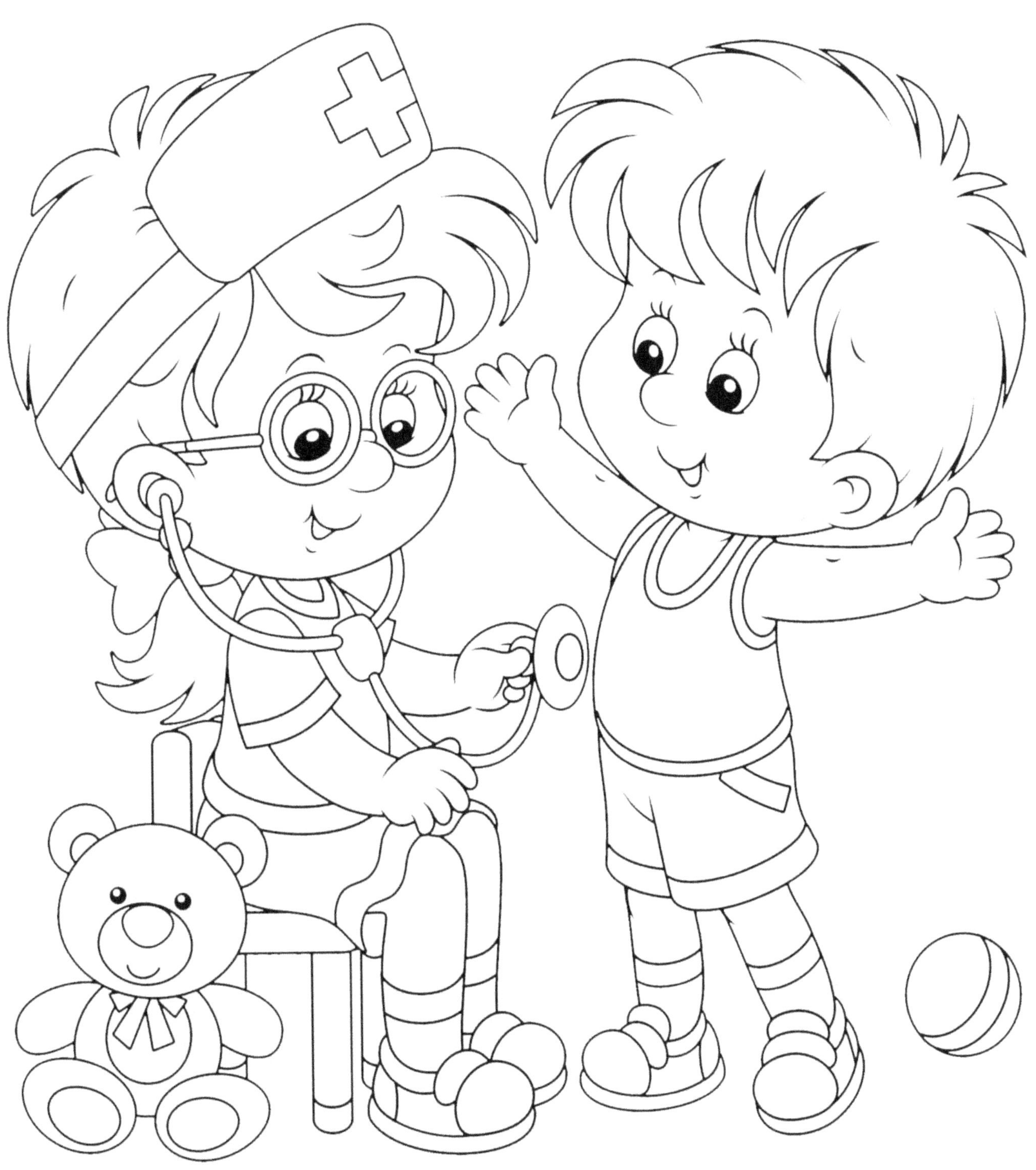

Test Your Color

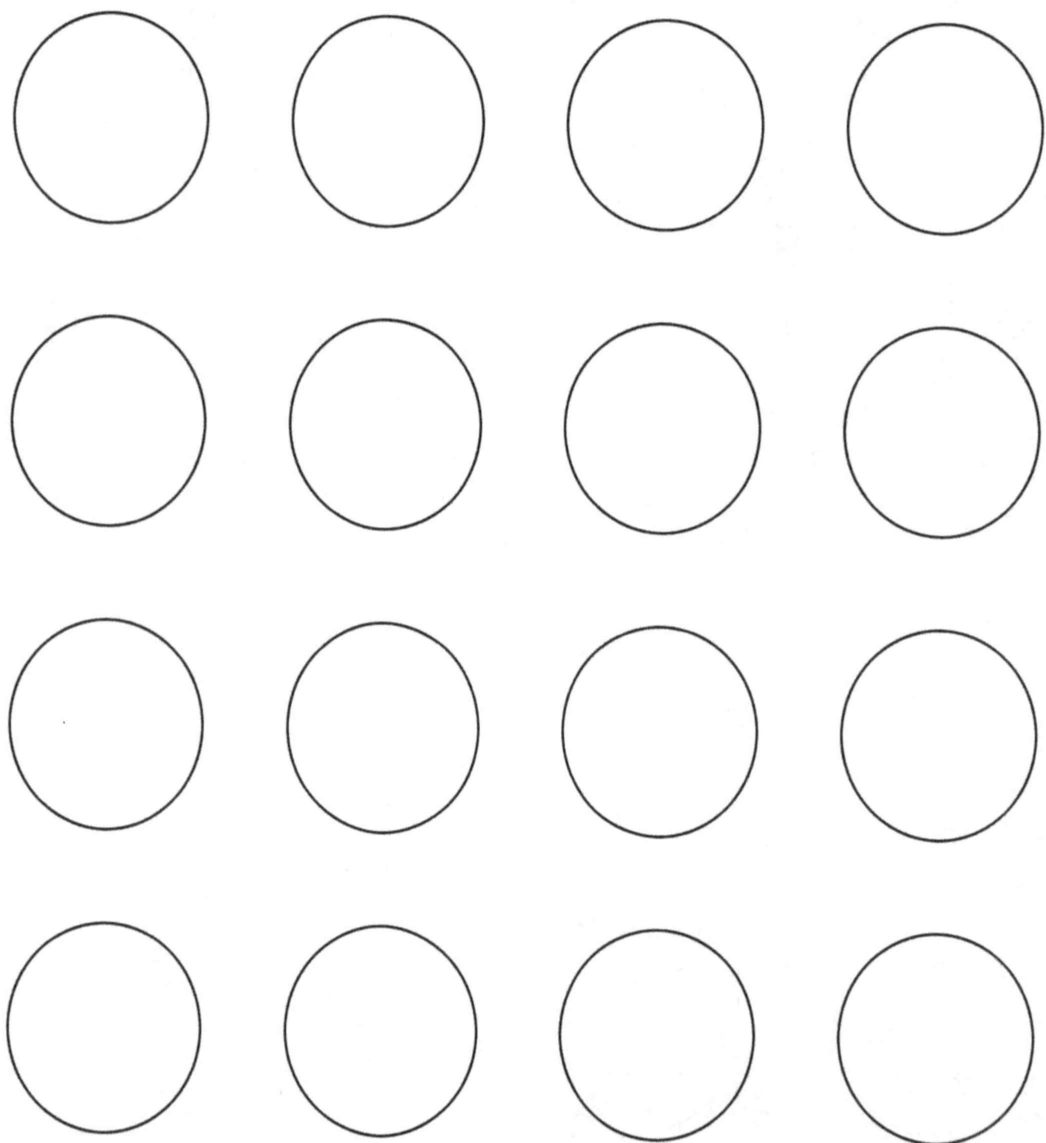

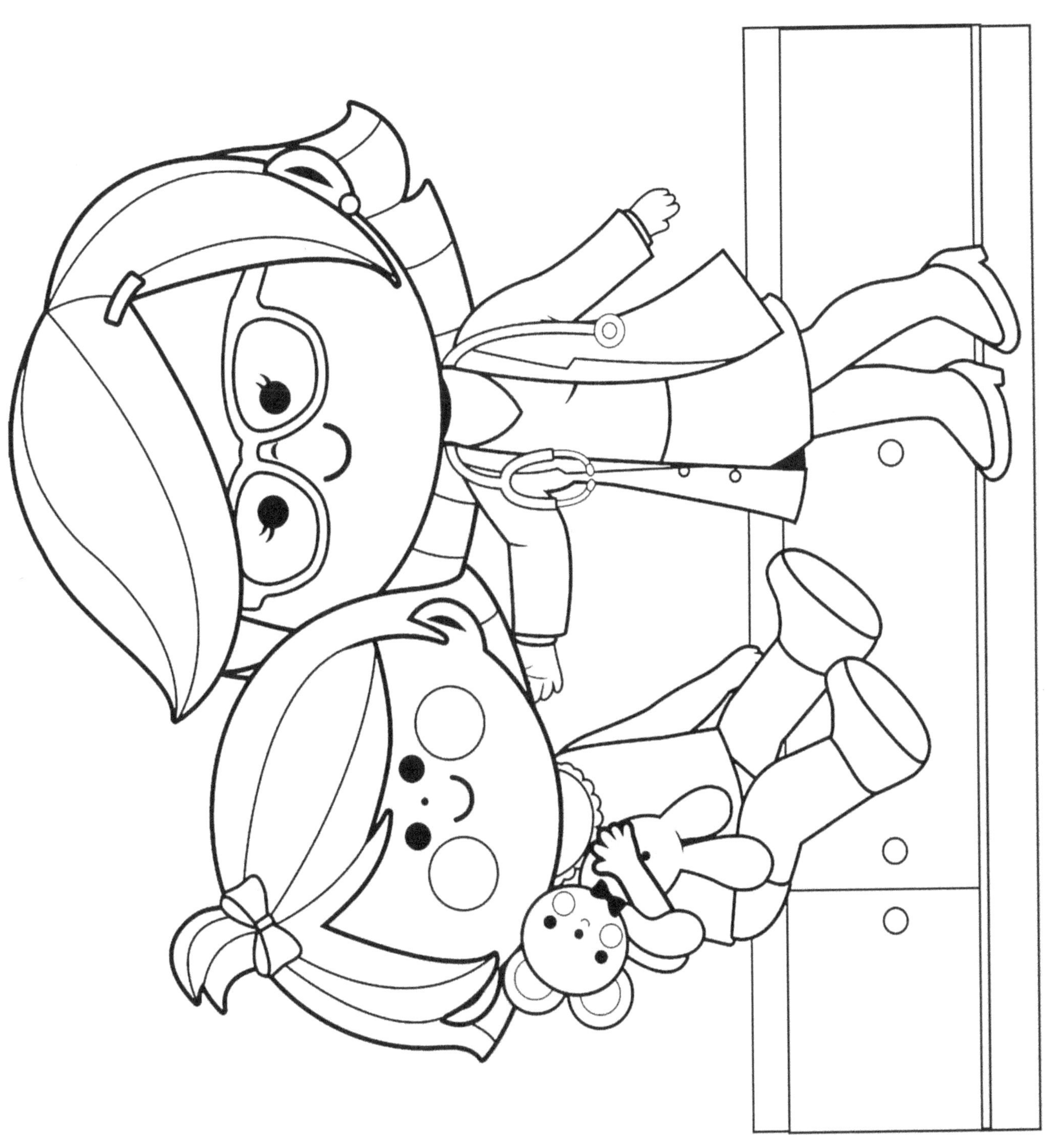

Test Your Color

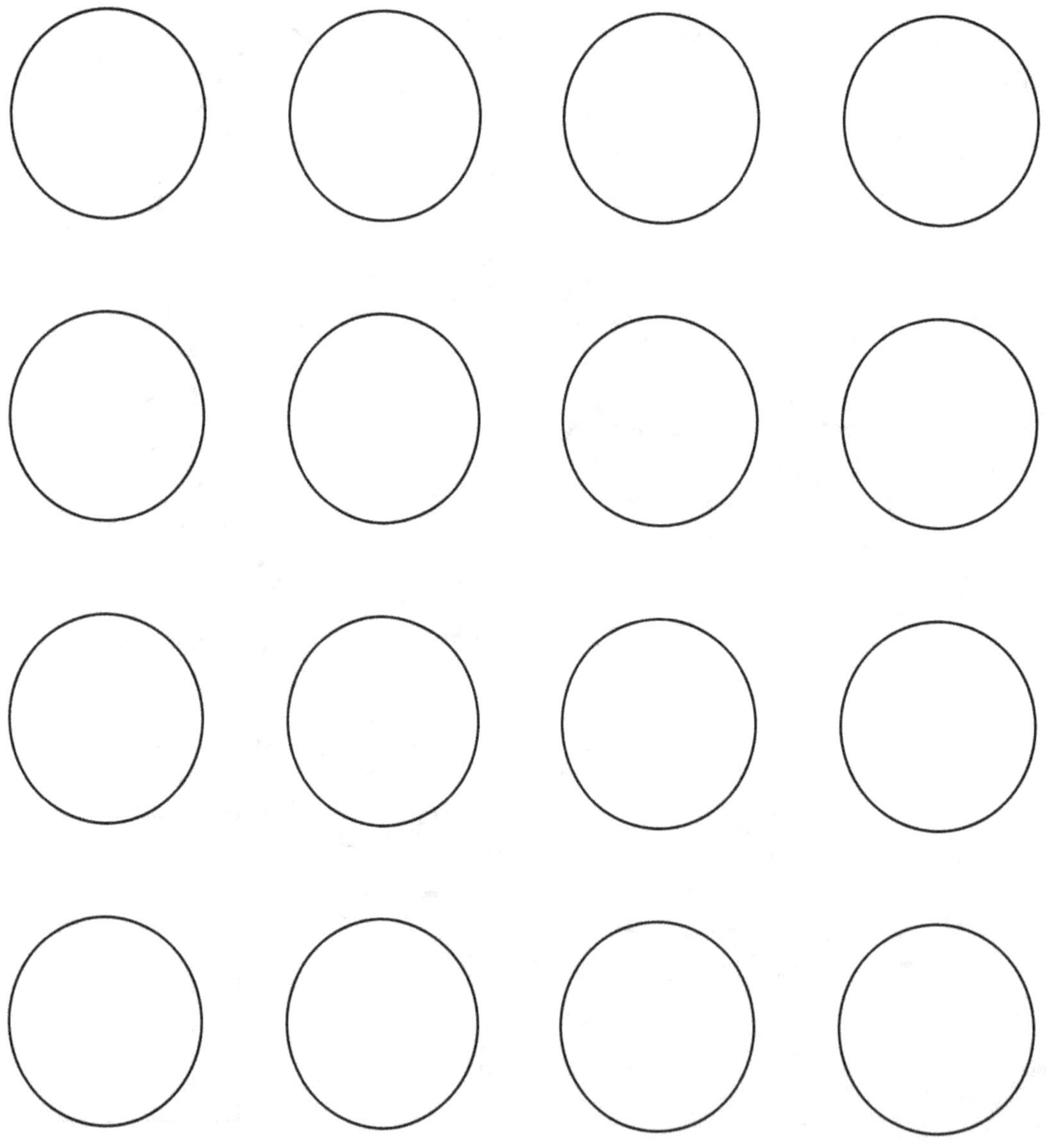

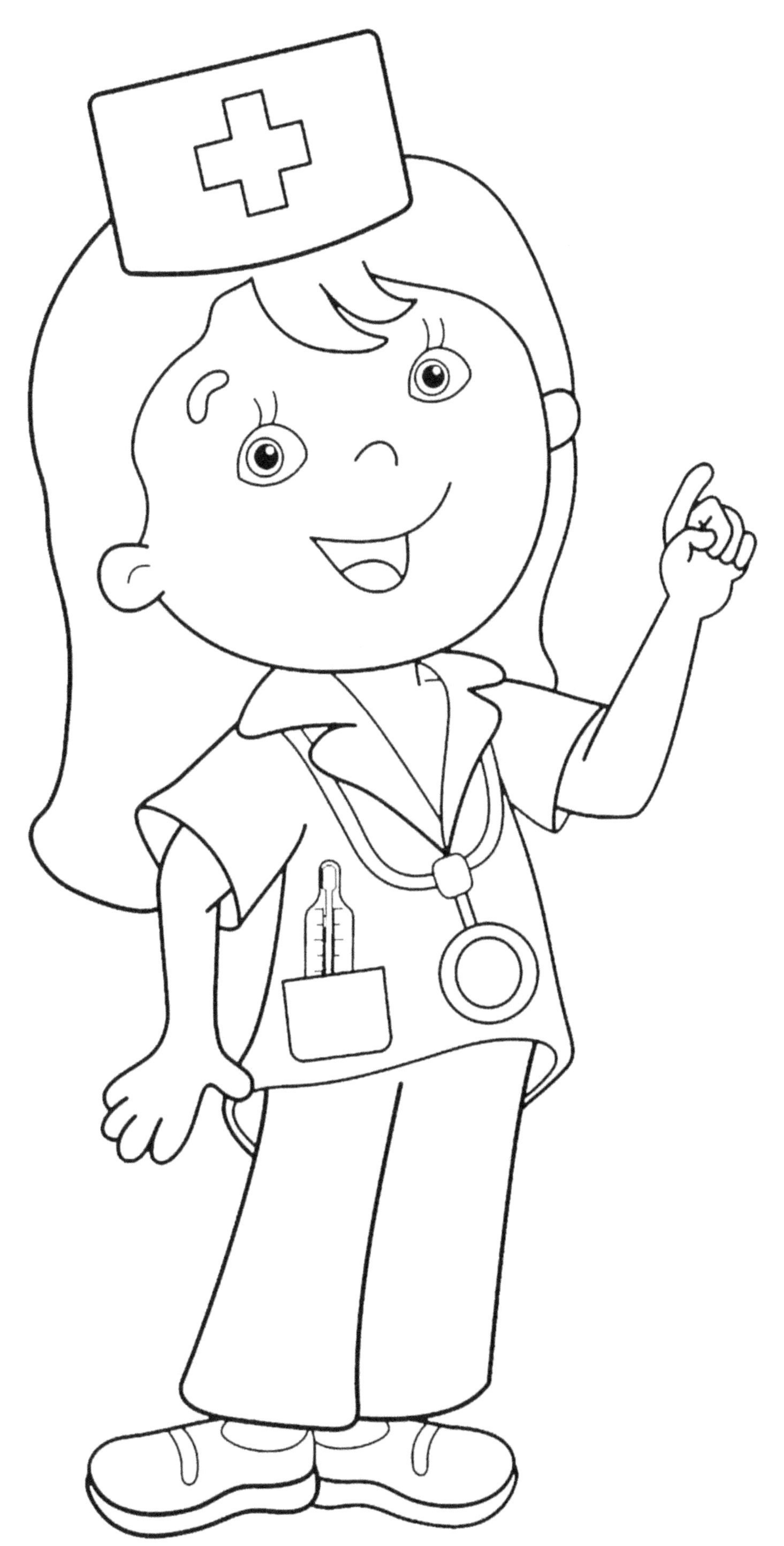

Test Your Color

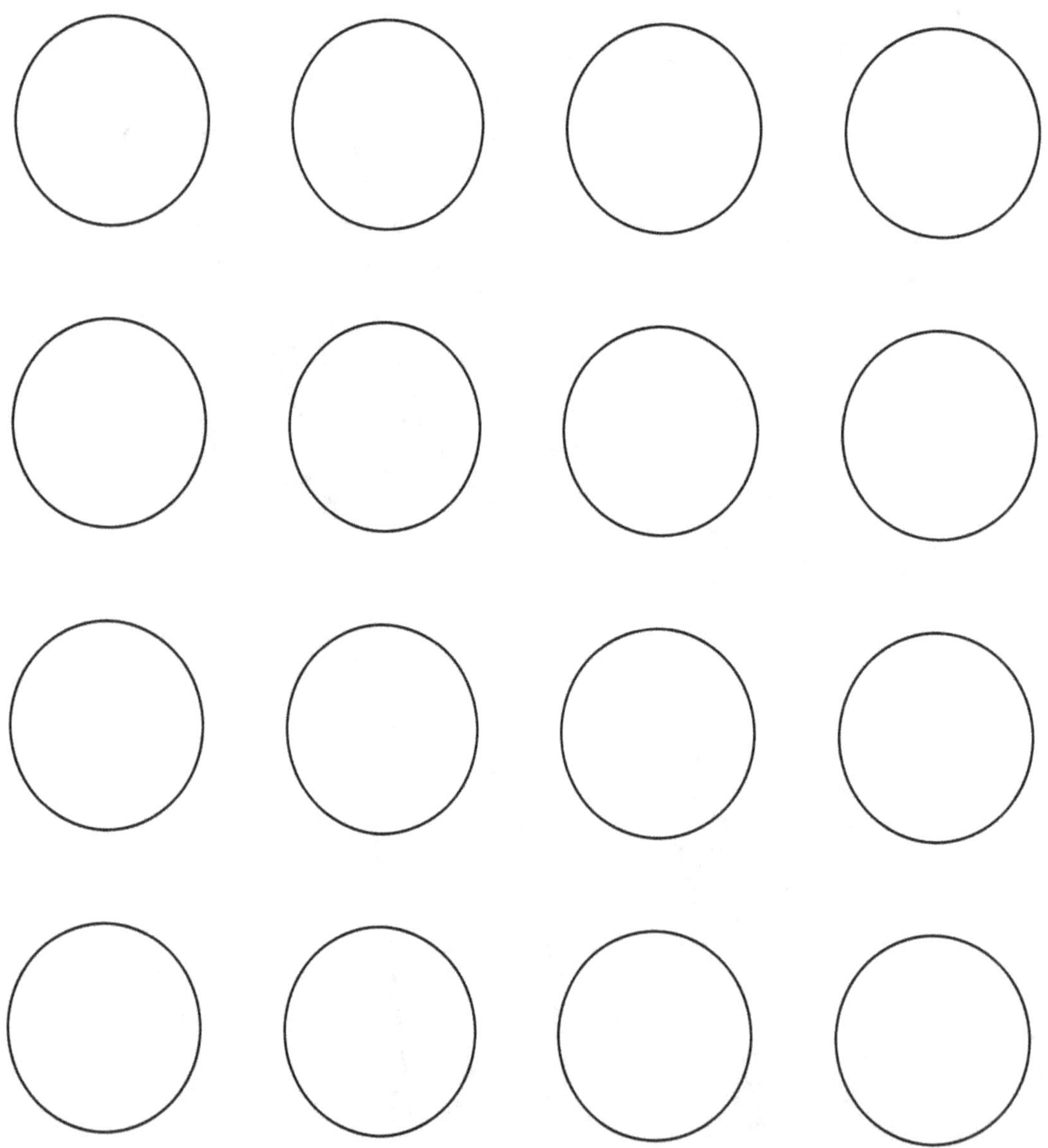

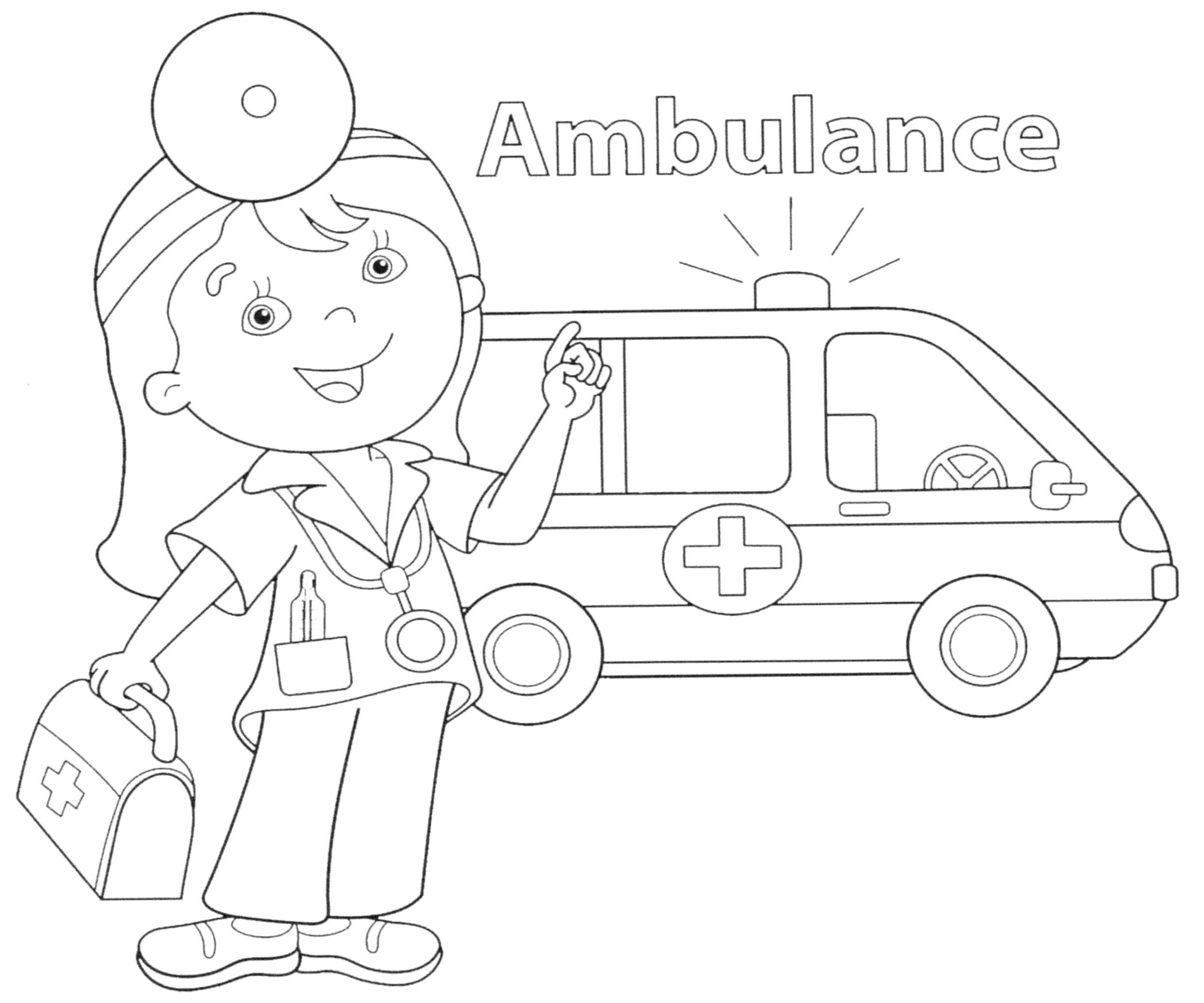

Ambulance

Test Your Color

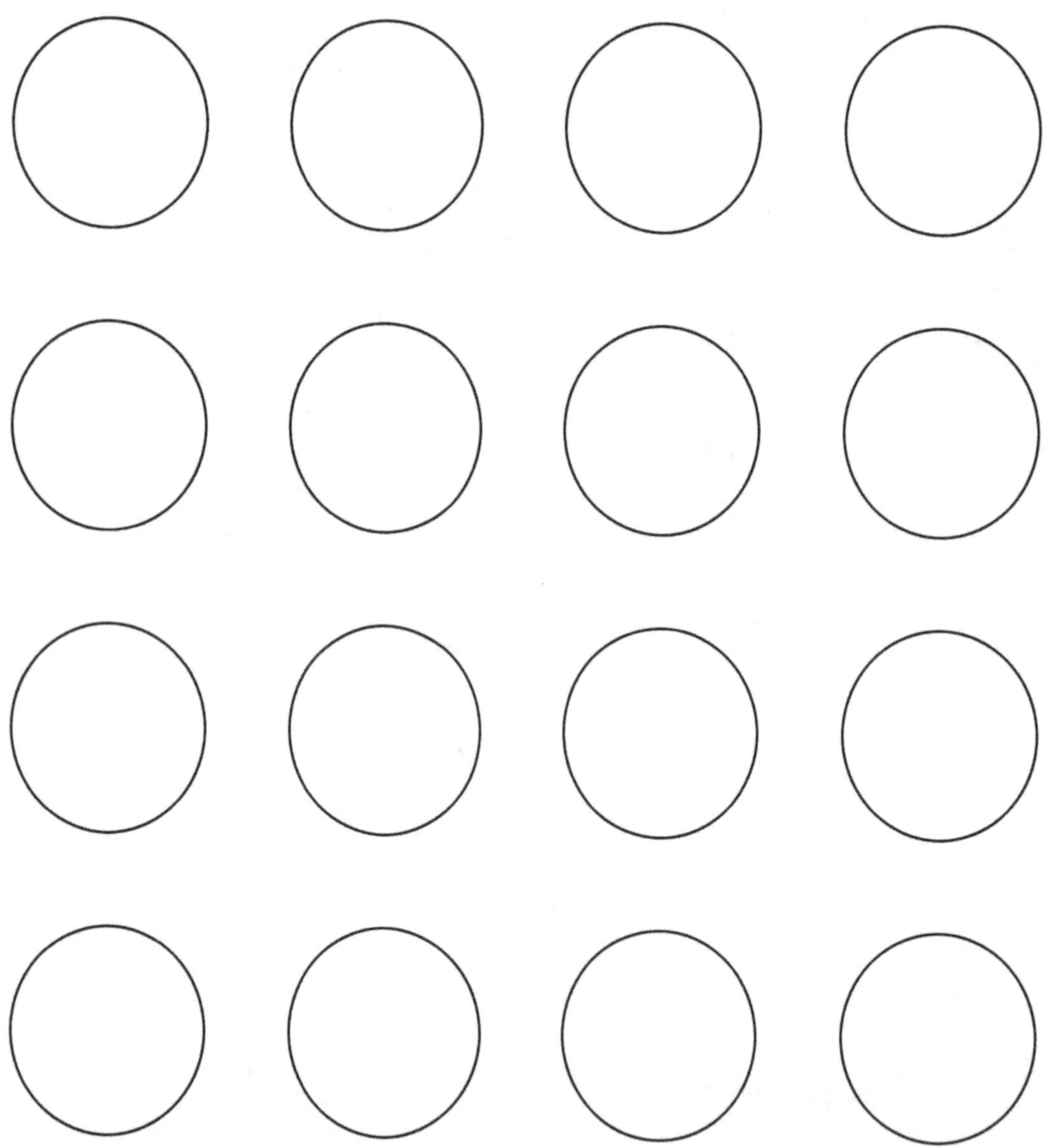

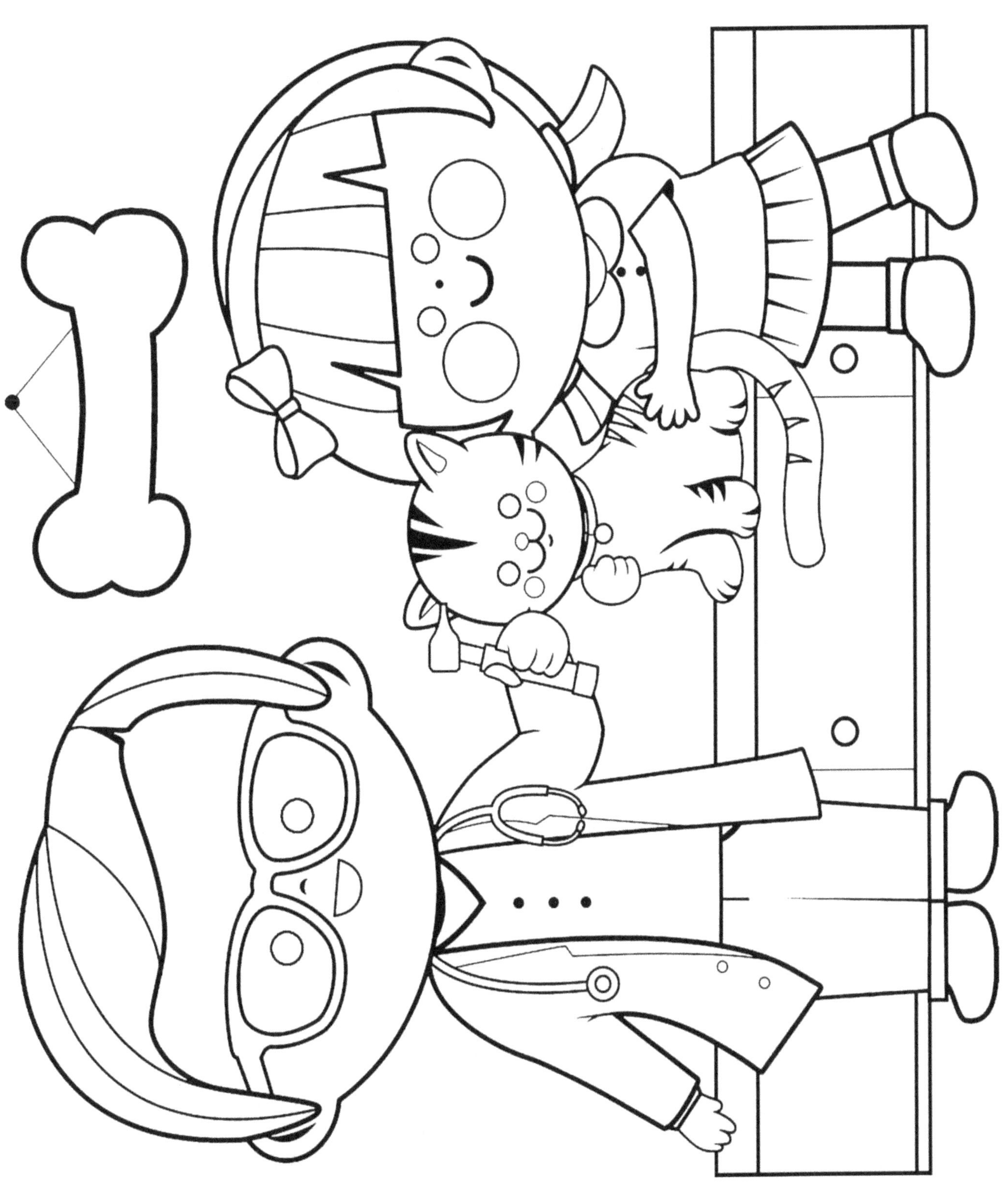

Test Your Color

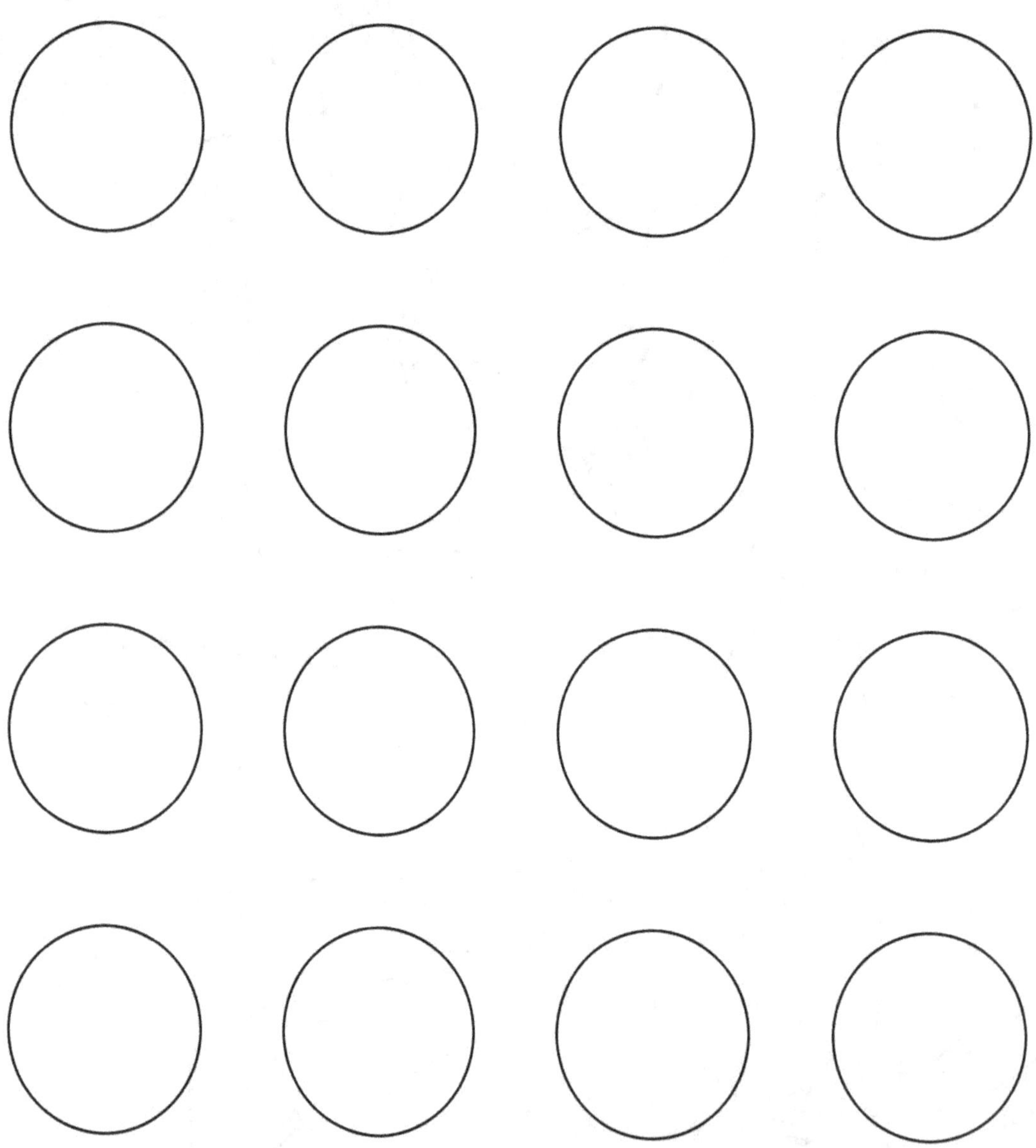

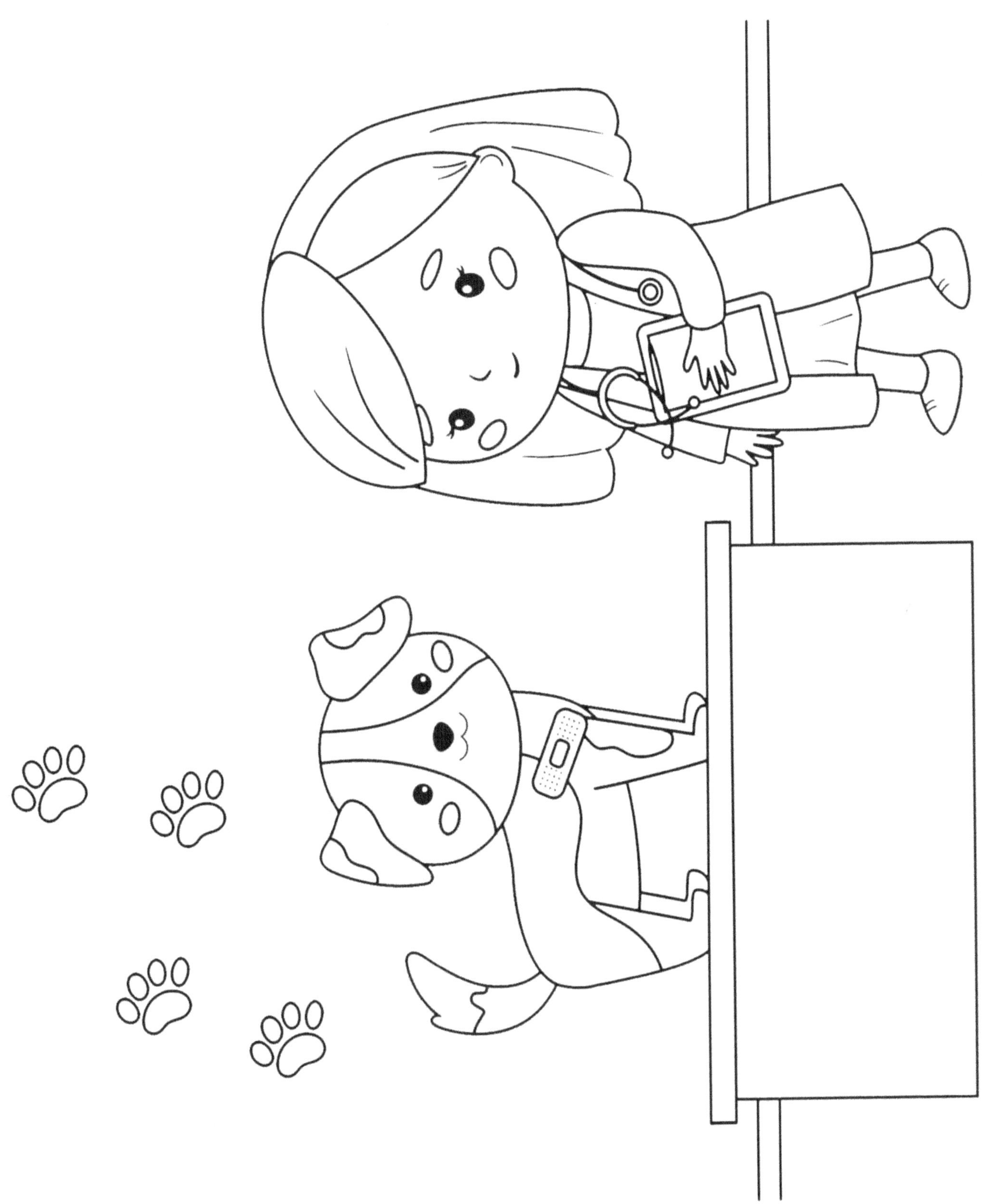

Test Your Color

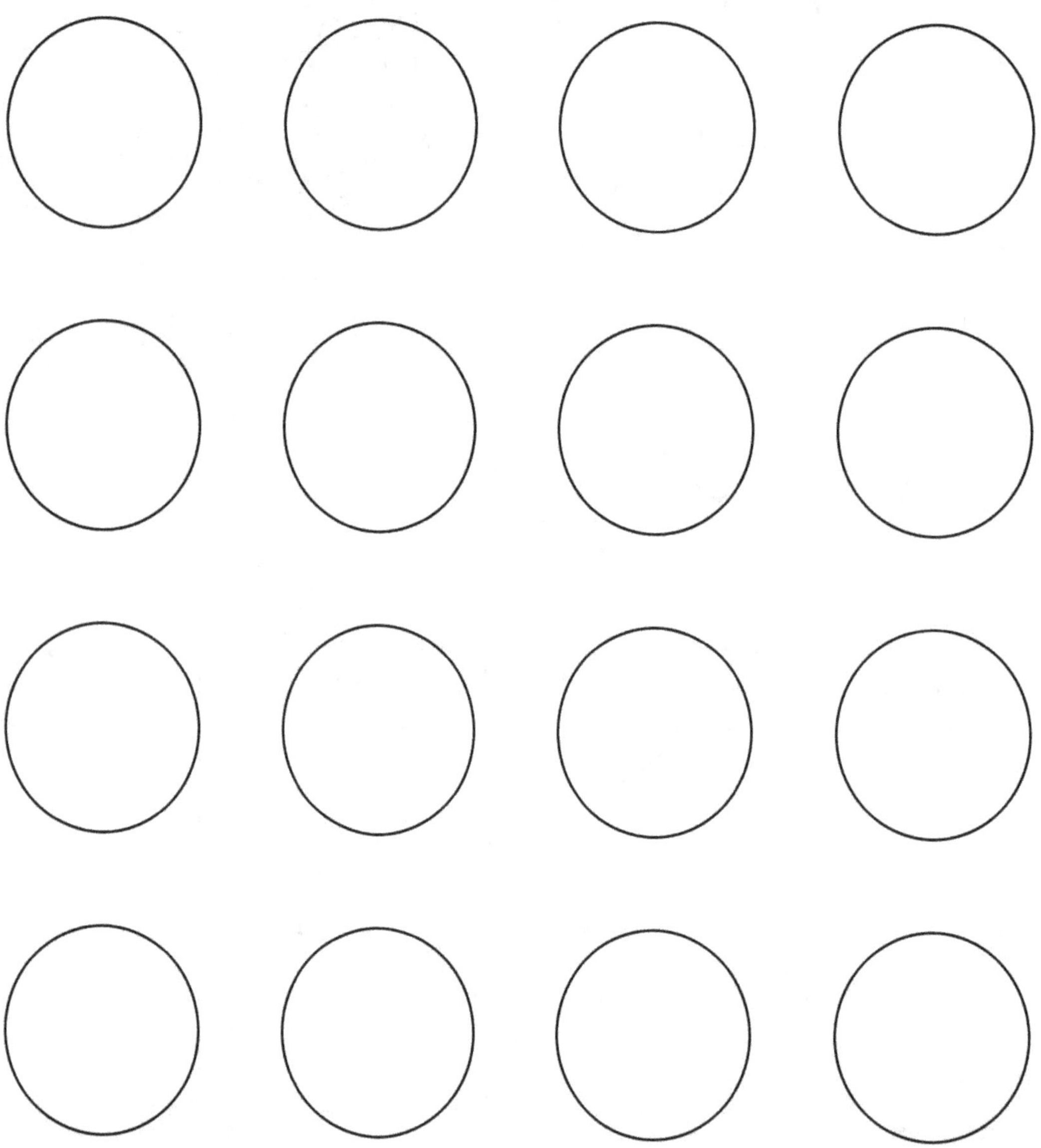

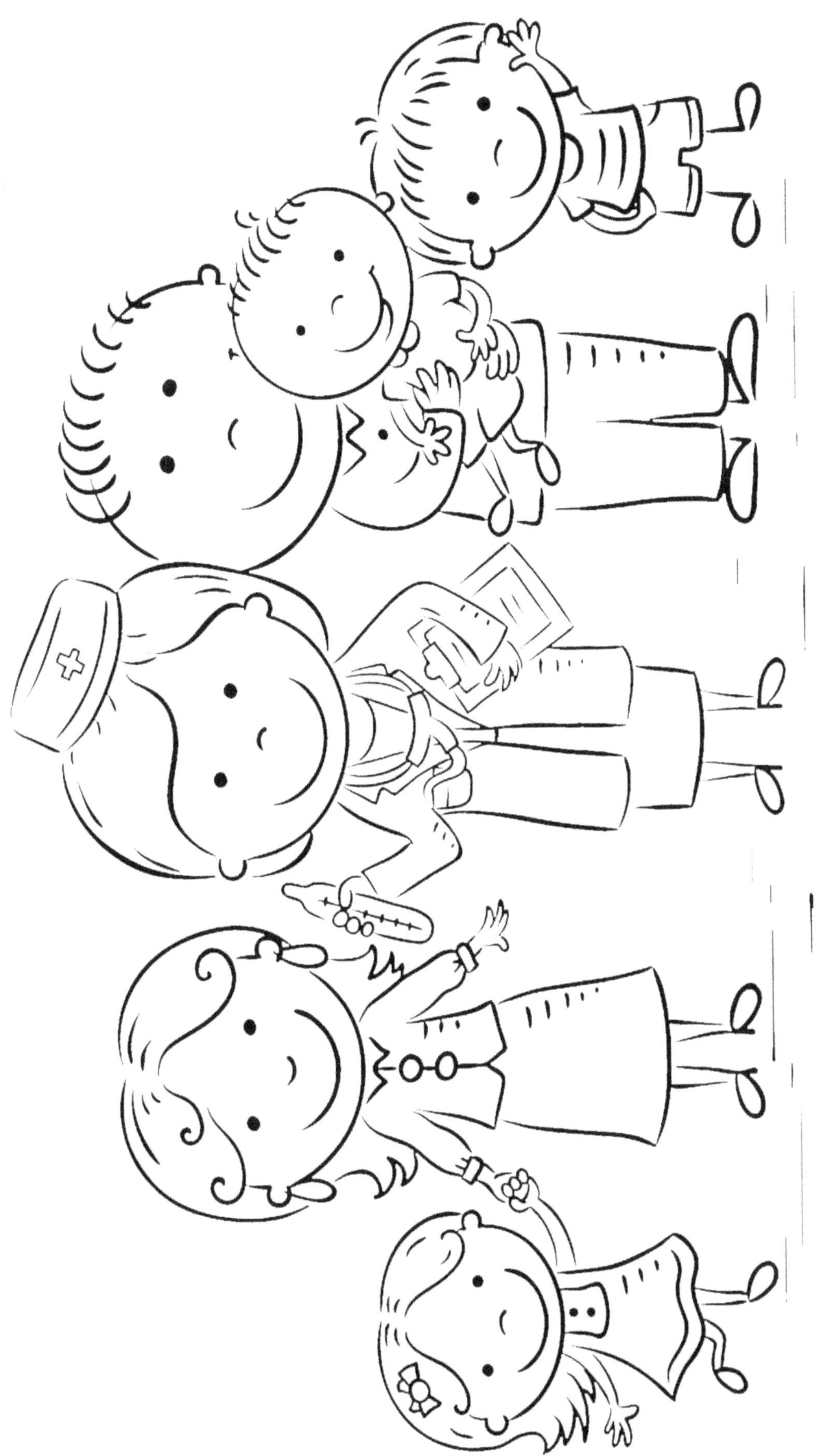

Test Your Color

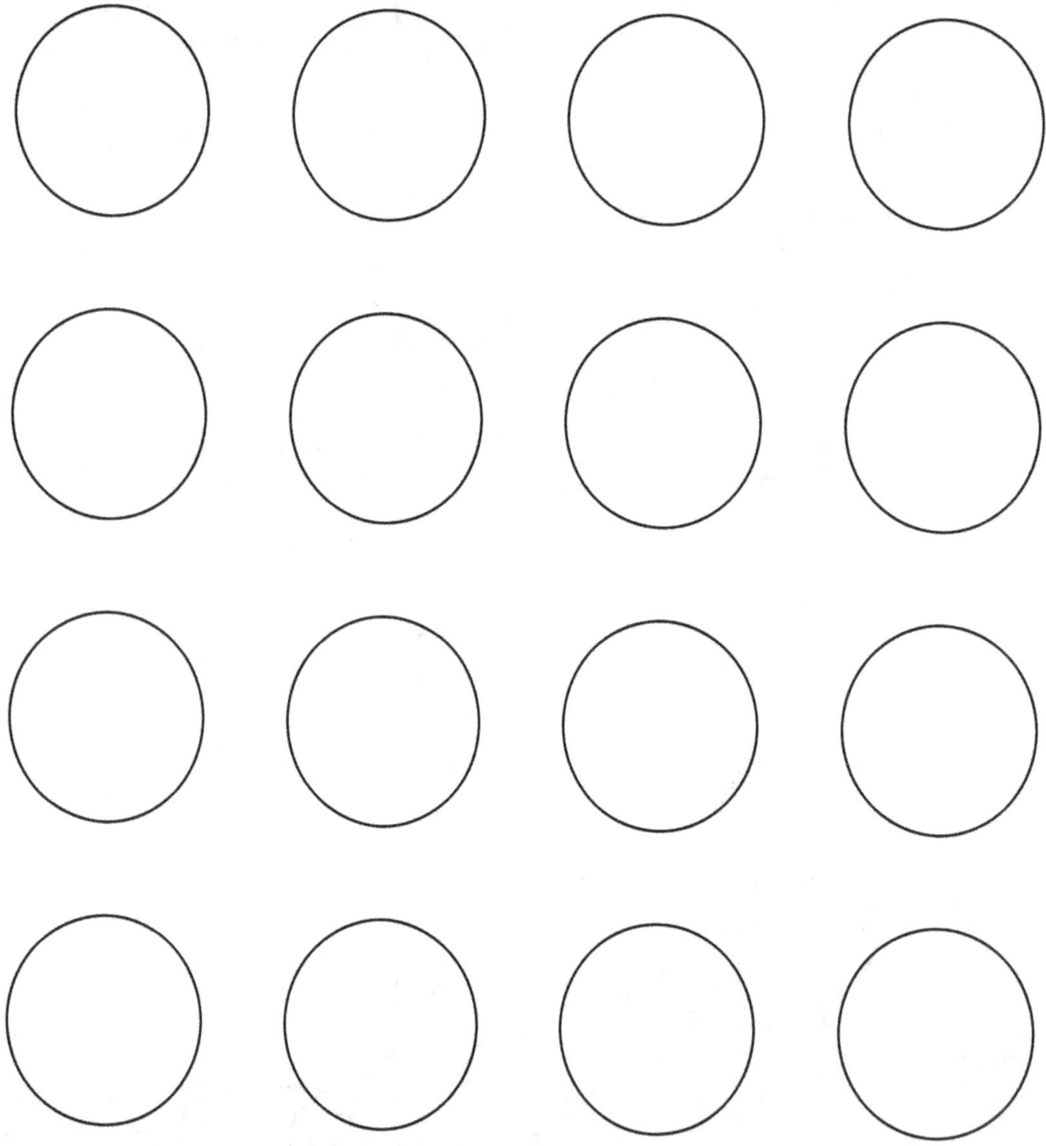

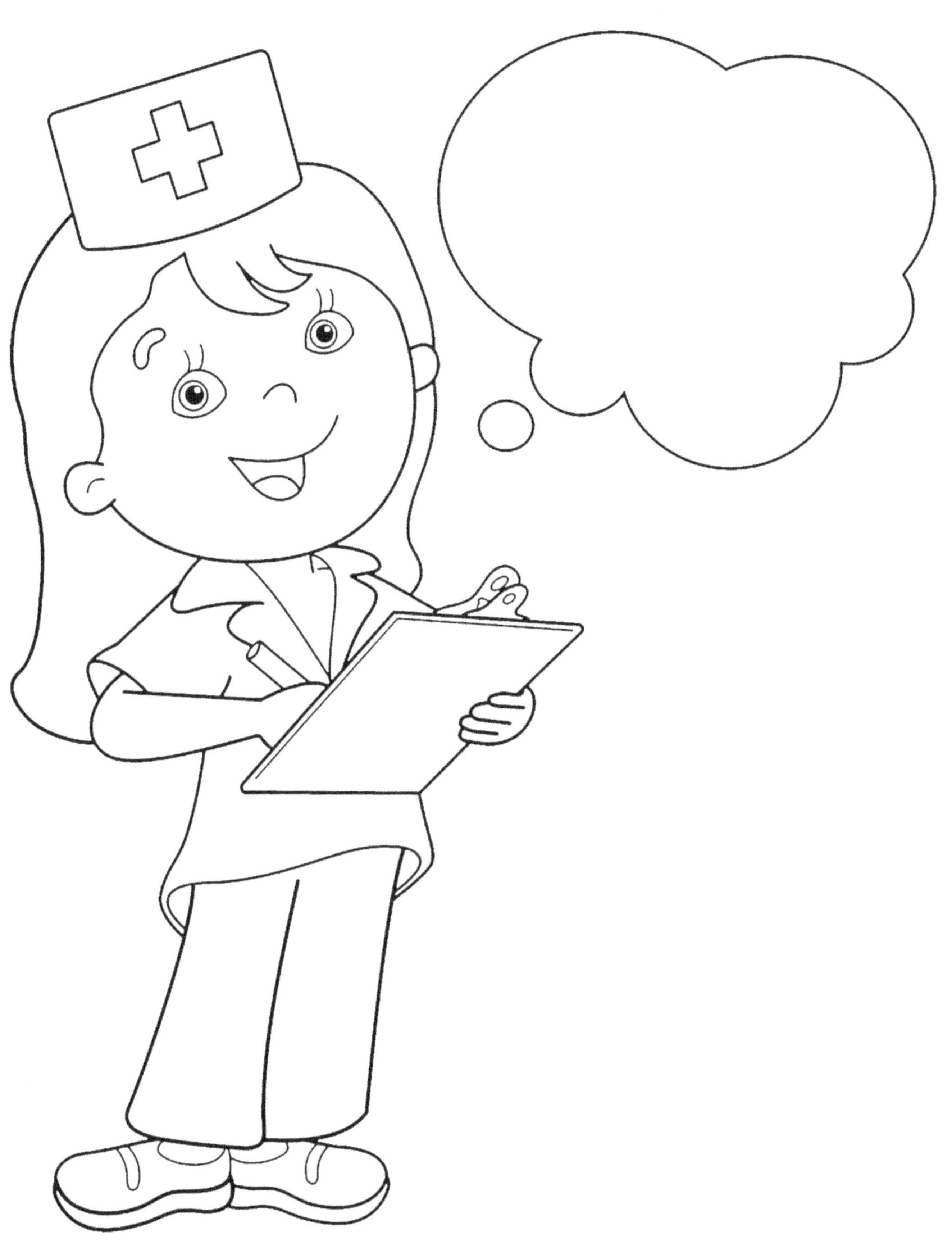

Test Your Color

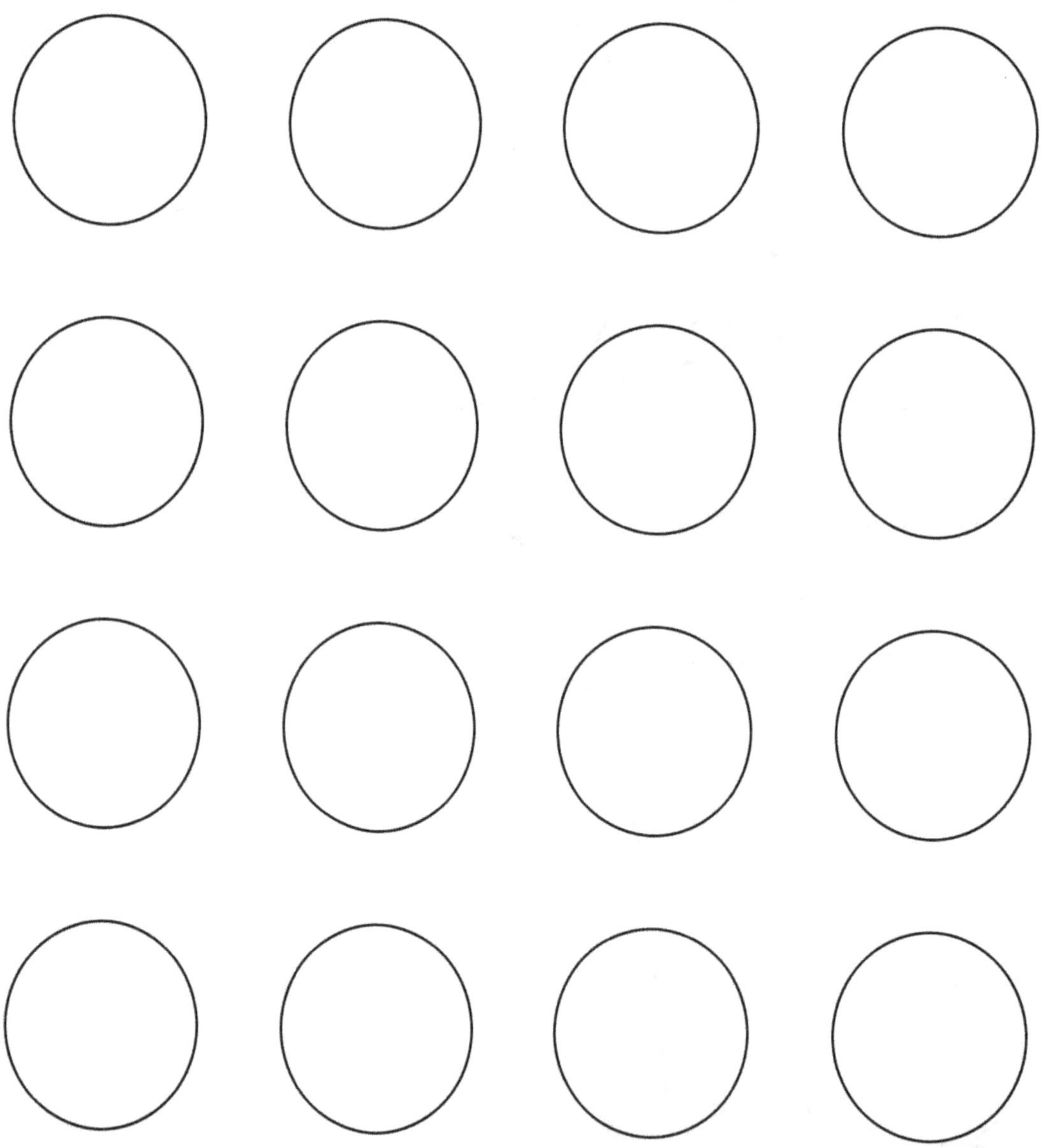

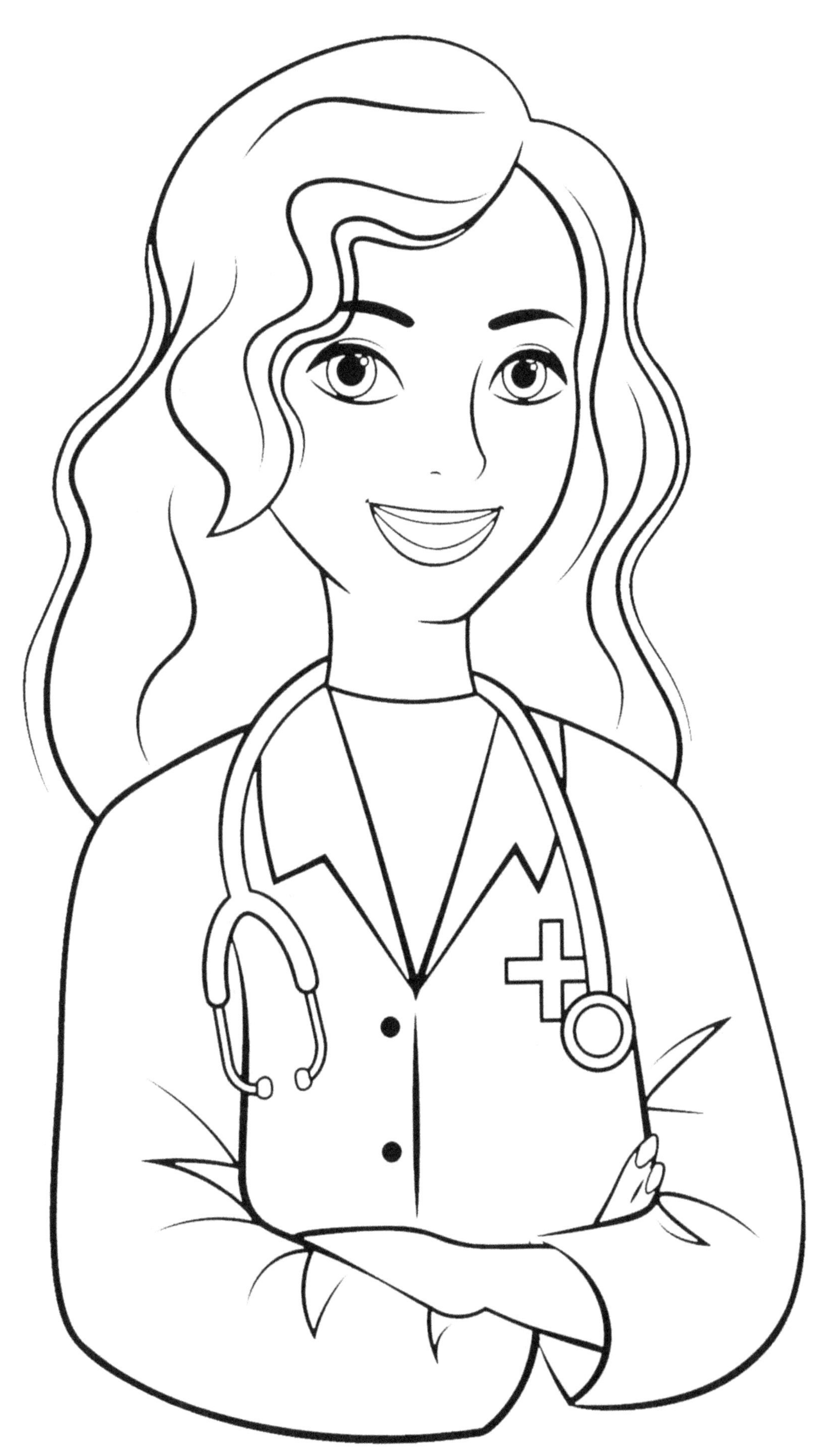

Test Your Color

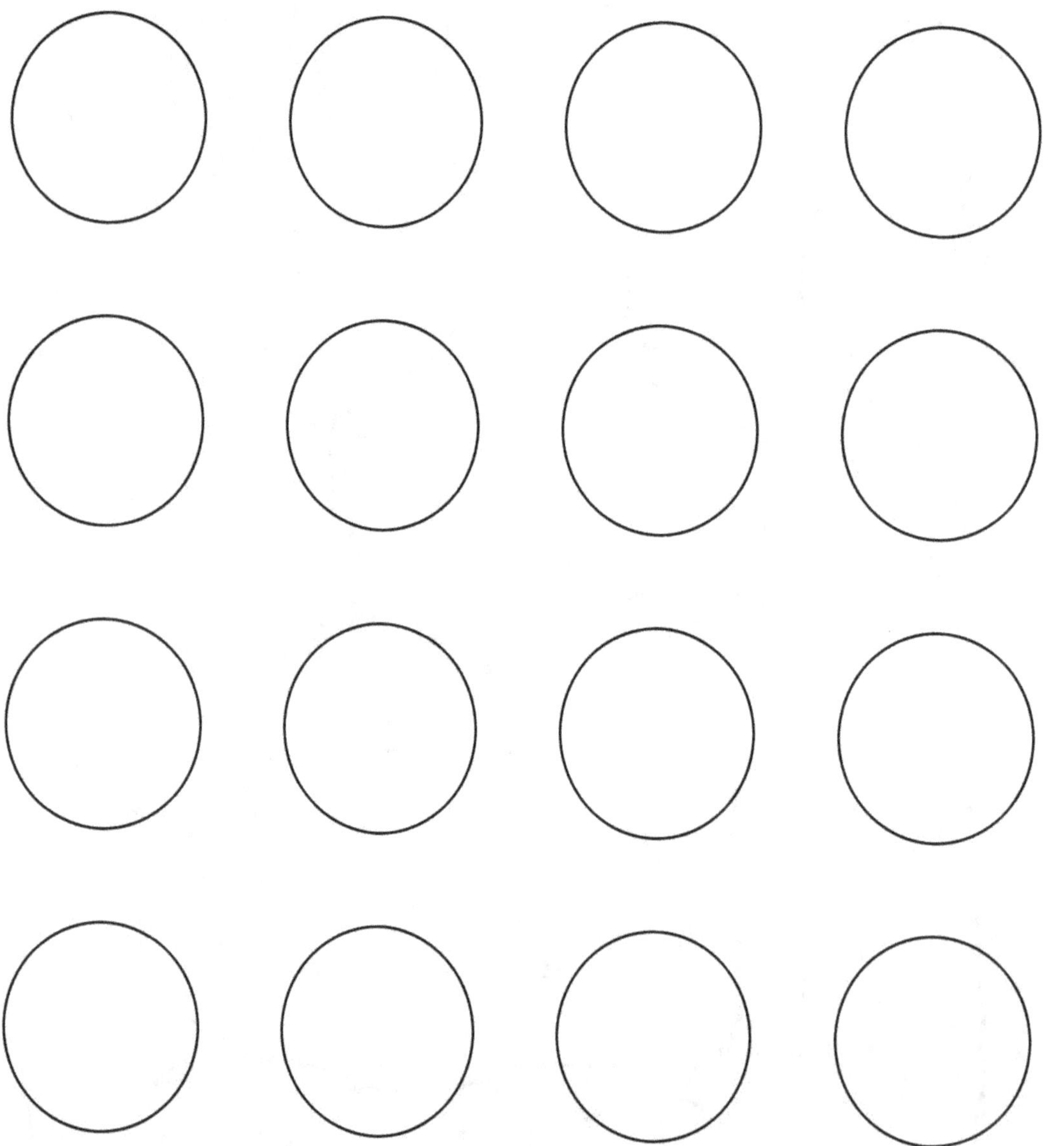

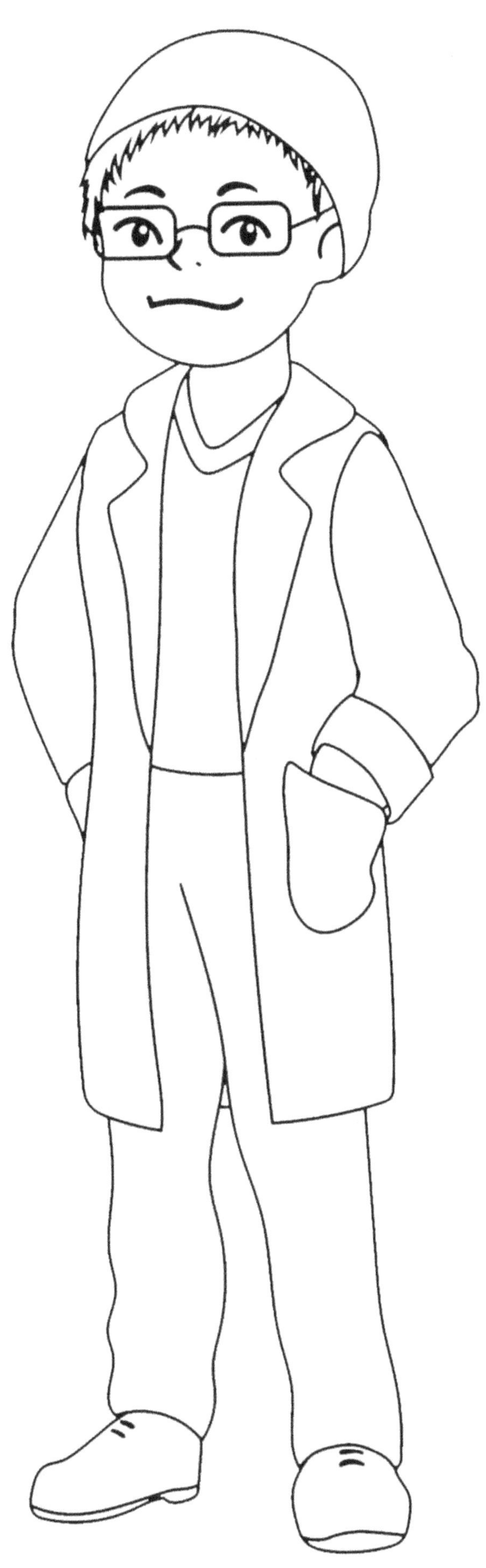

Test Your Color

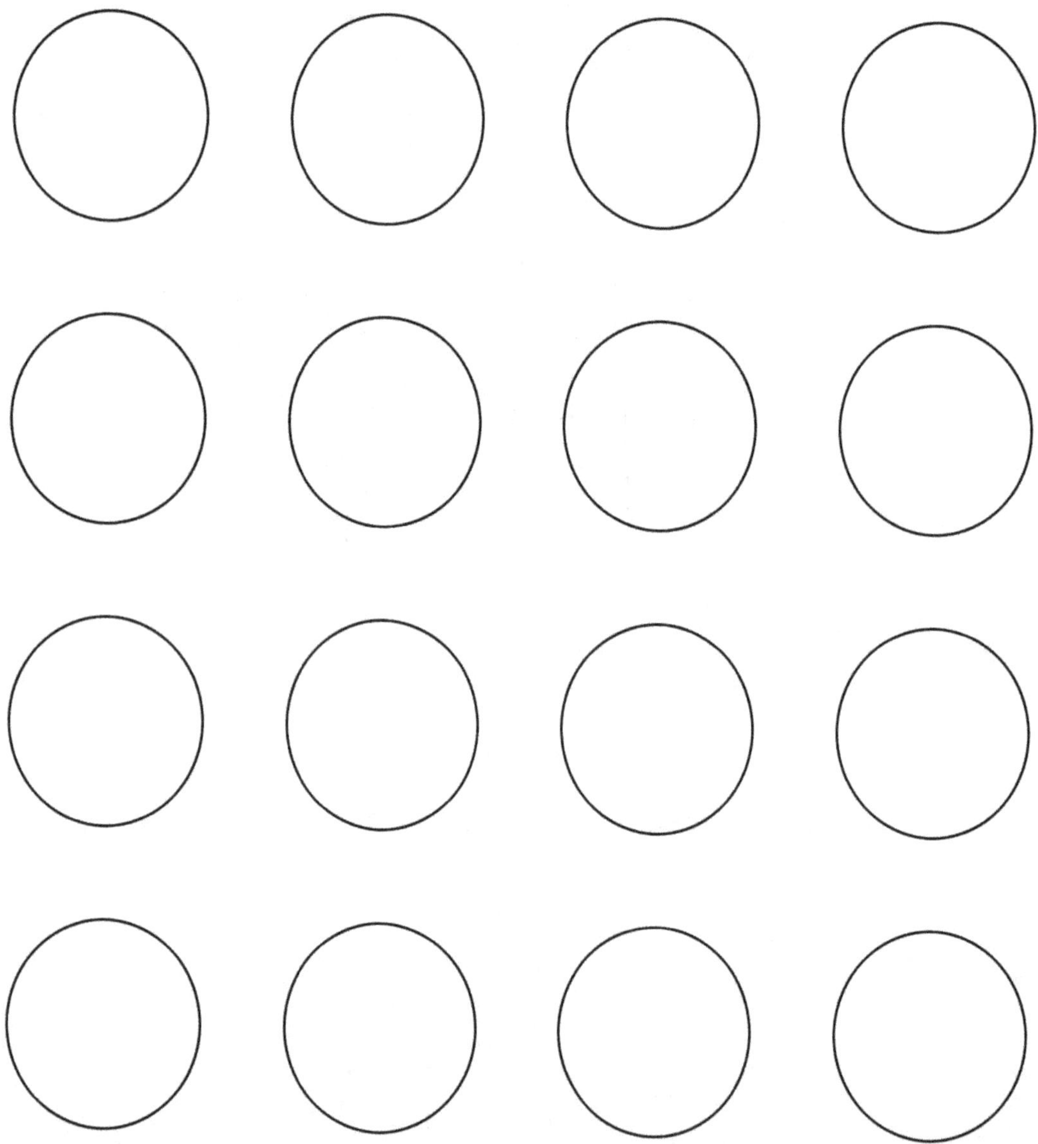

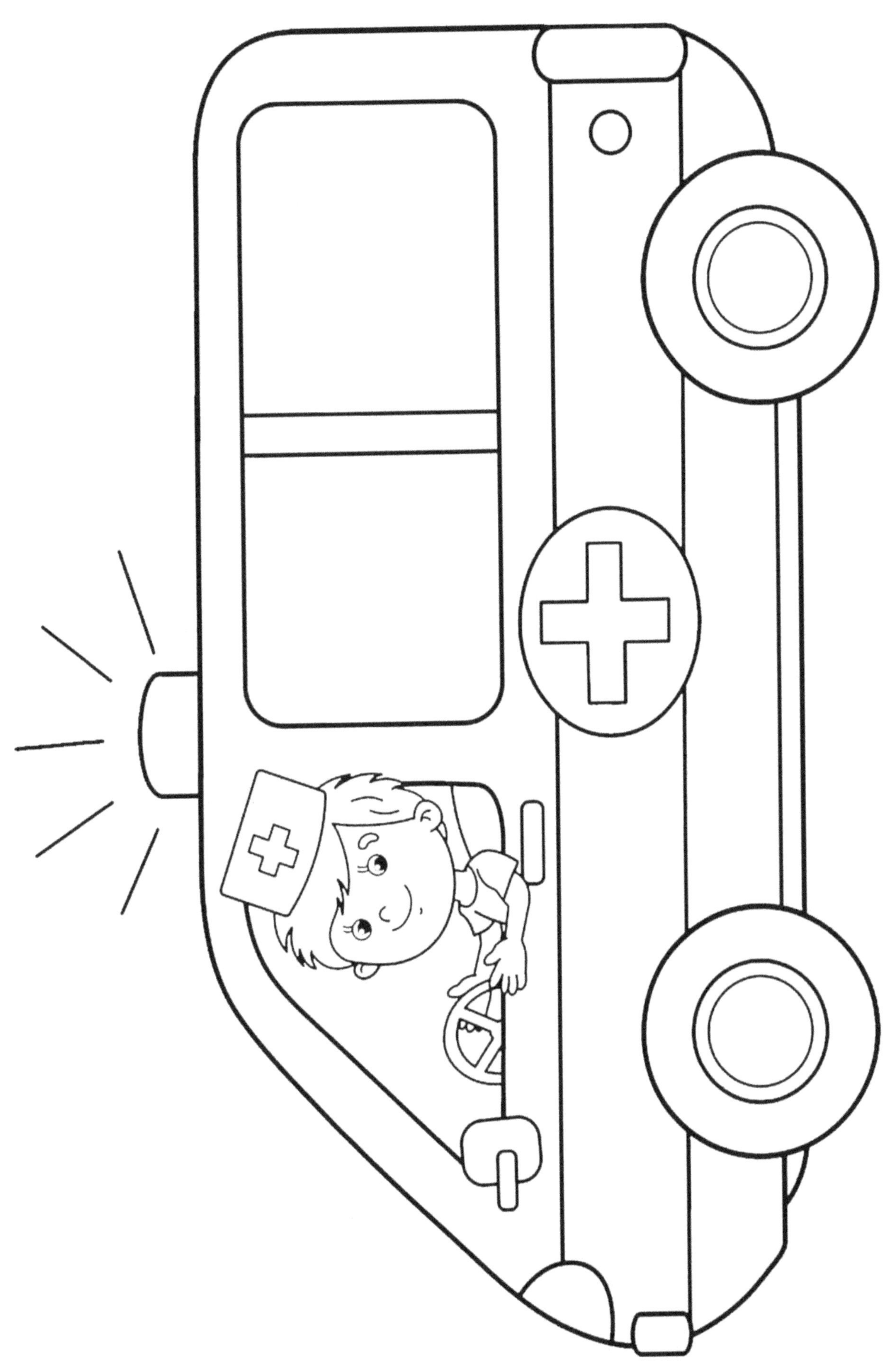

Test Your Color

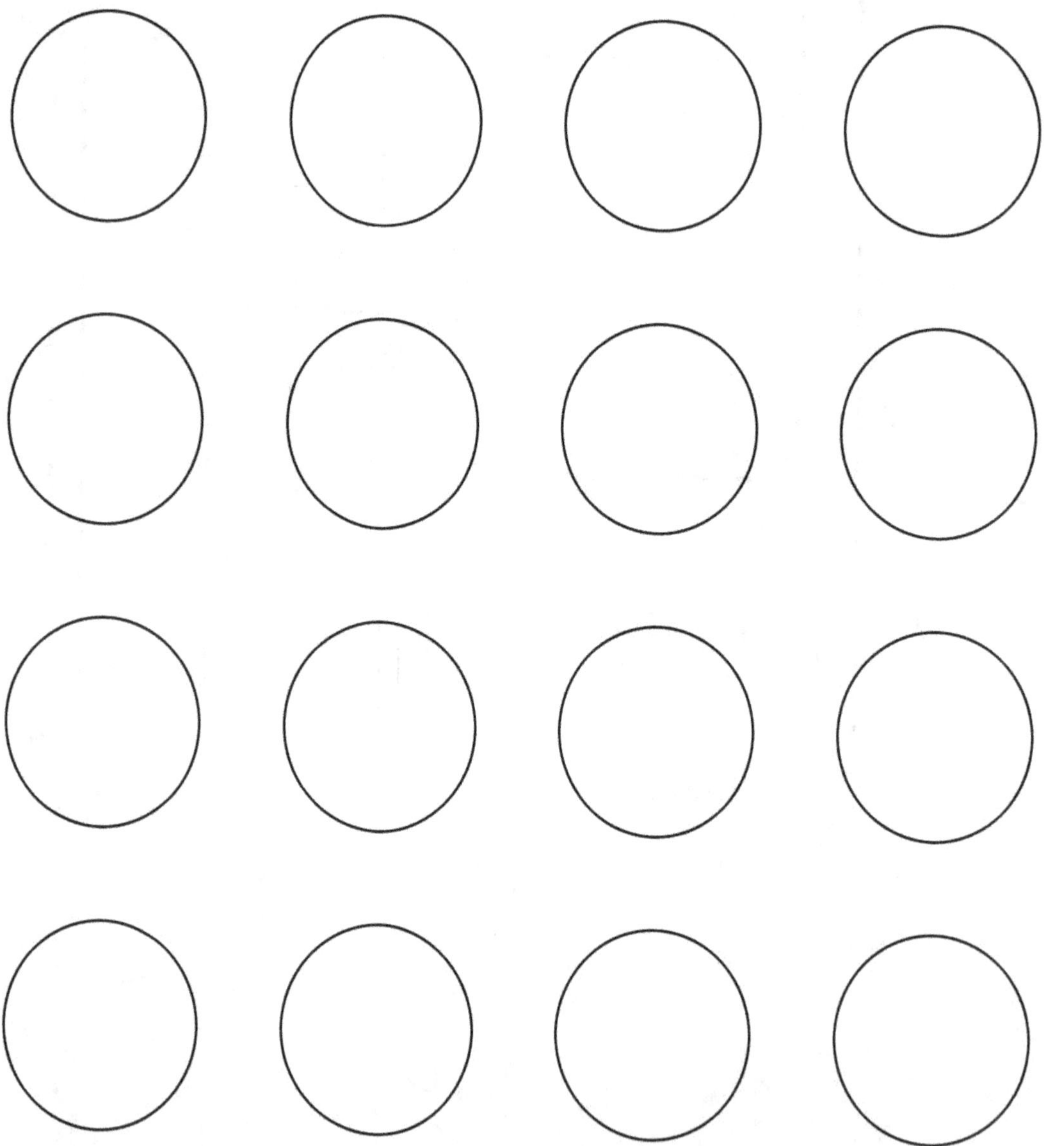

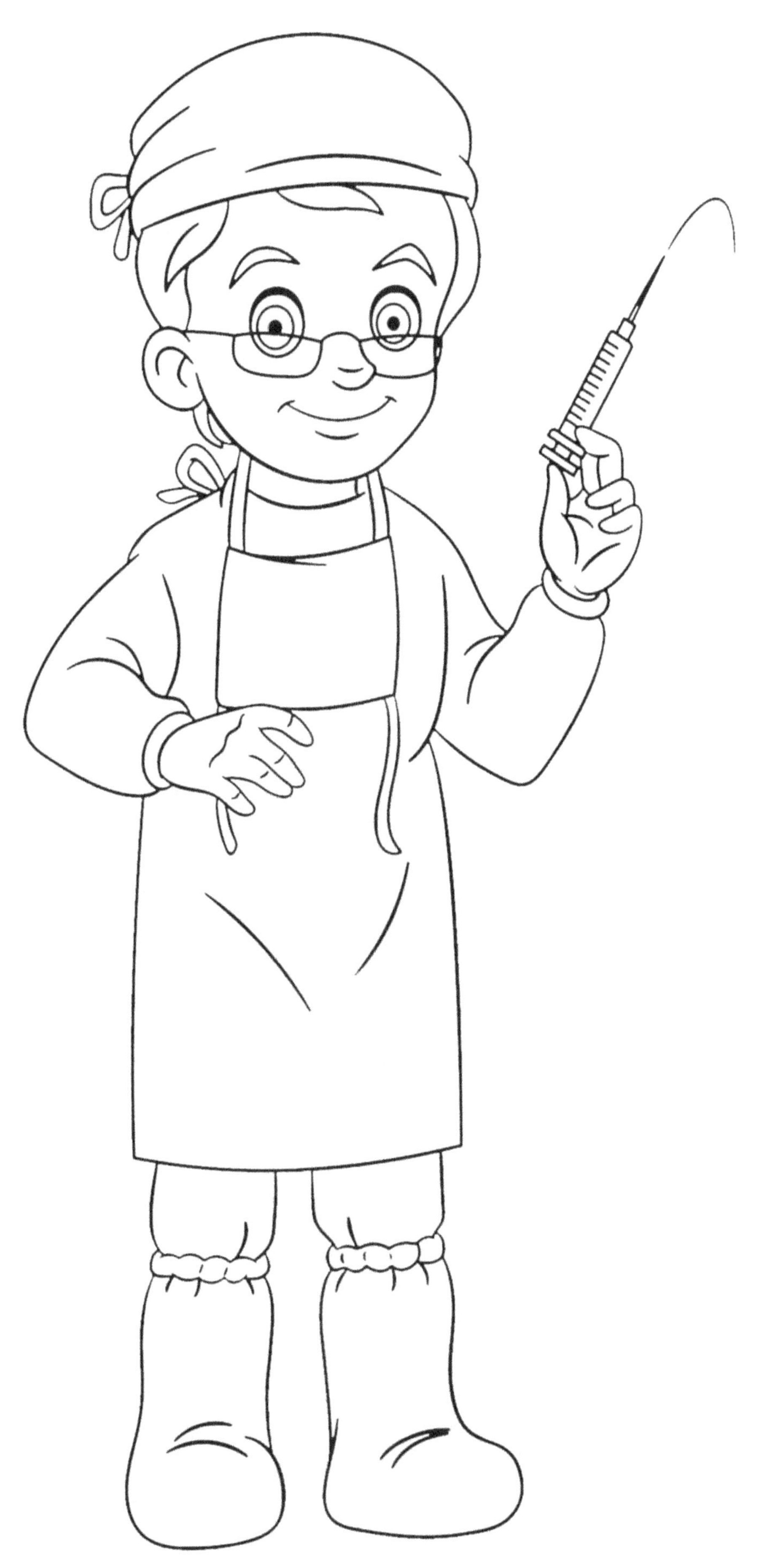

Test Your Color

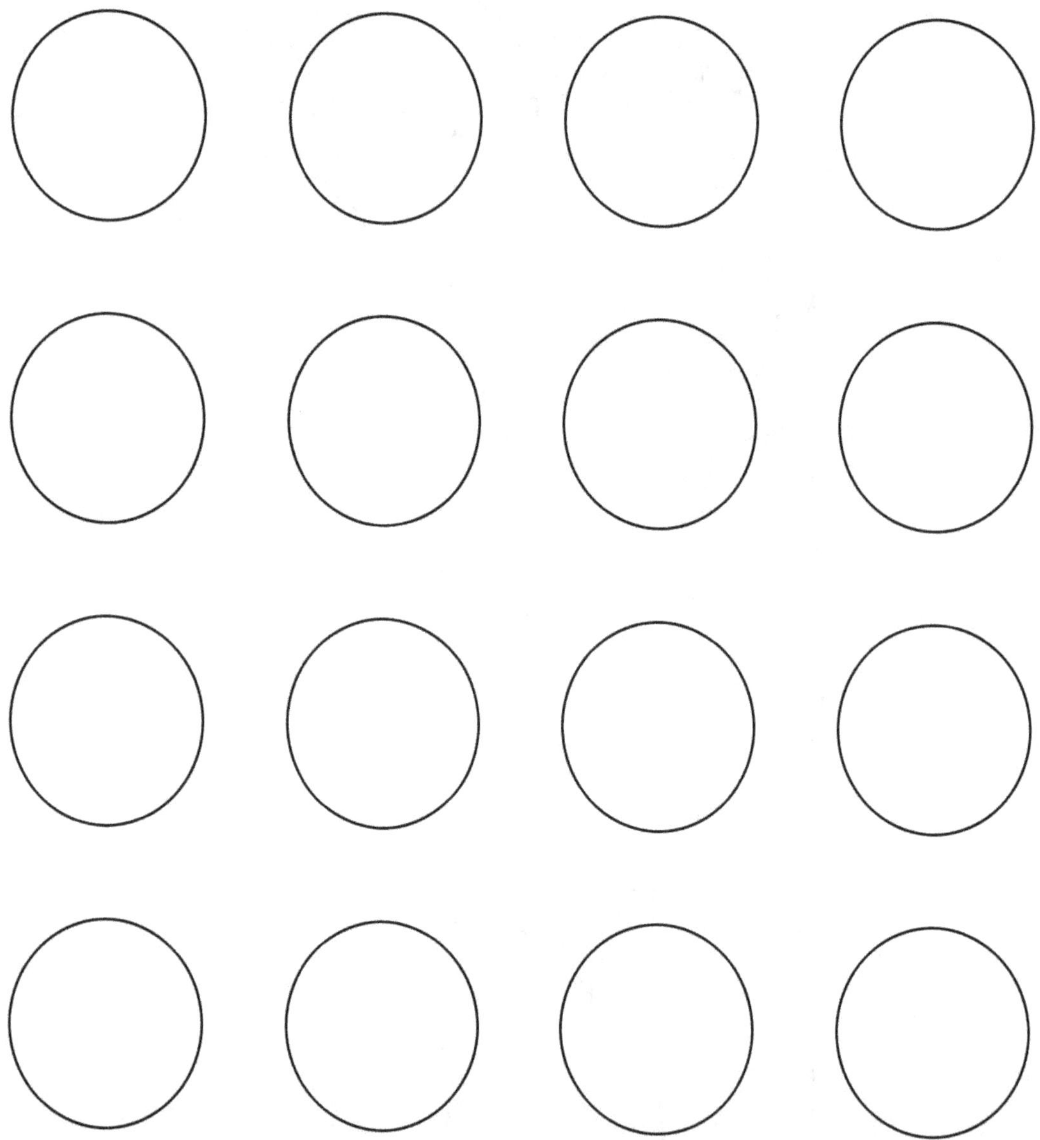

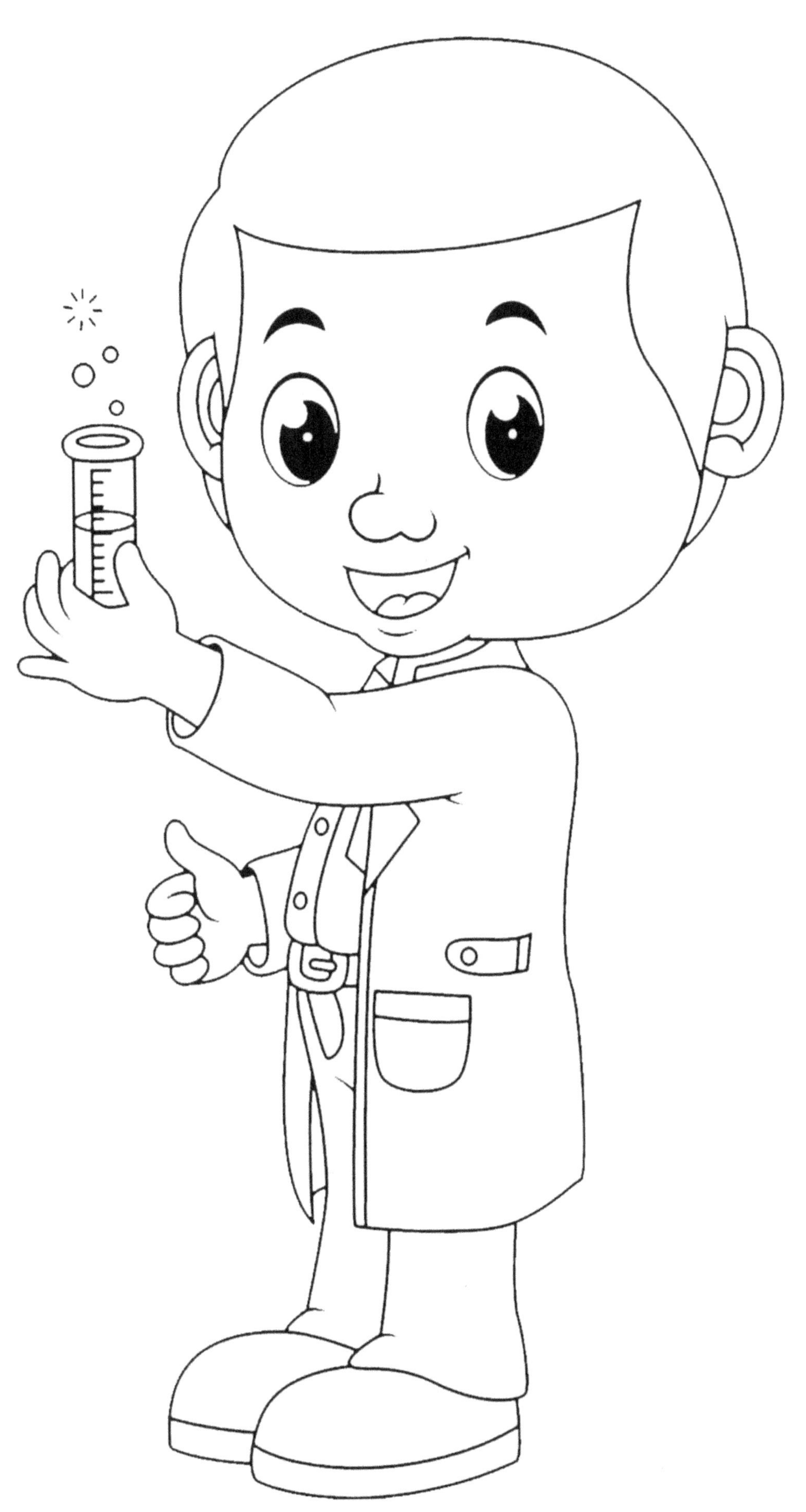

Test Your Color

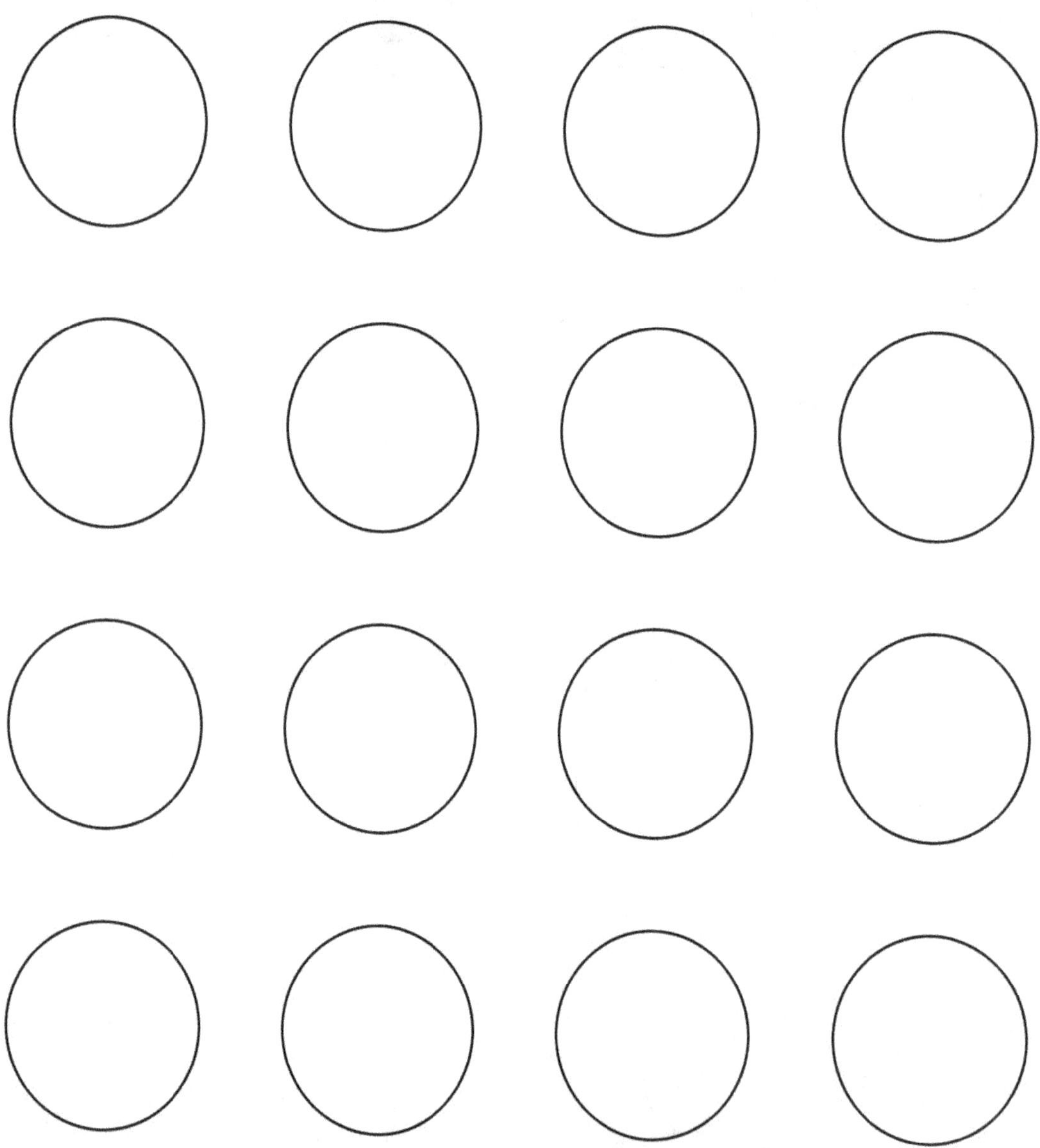

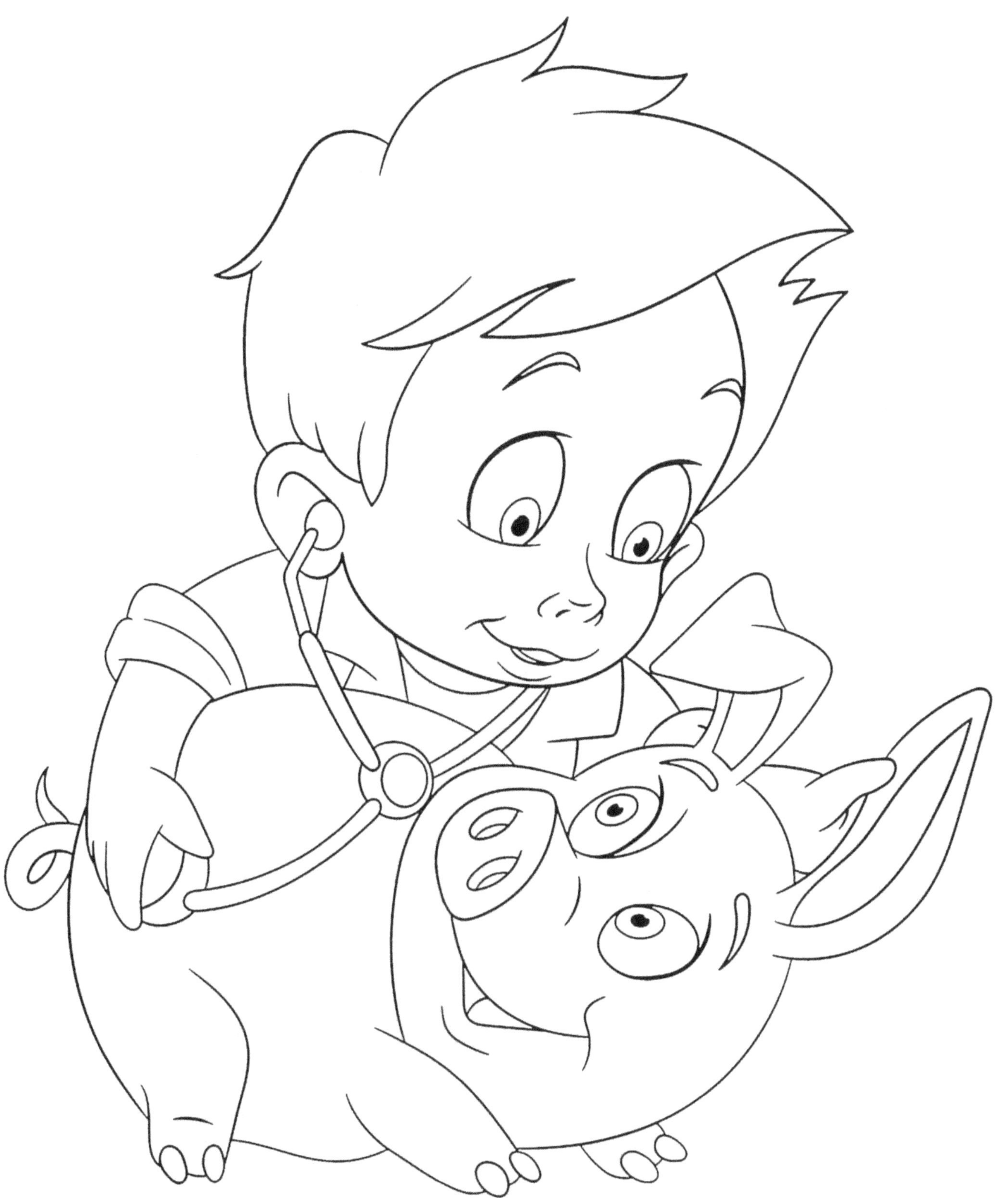

Test Your Color

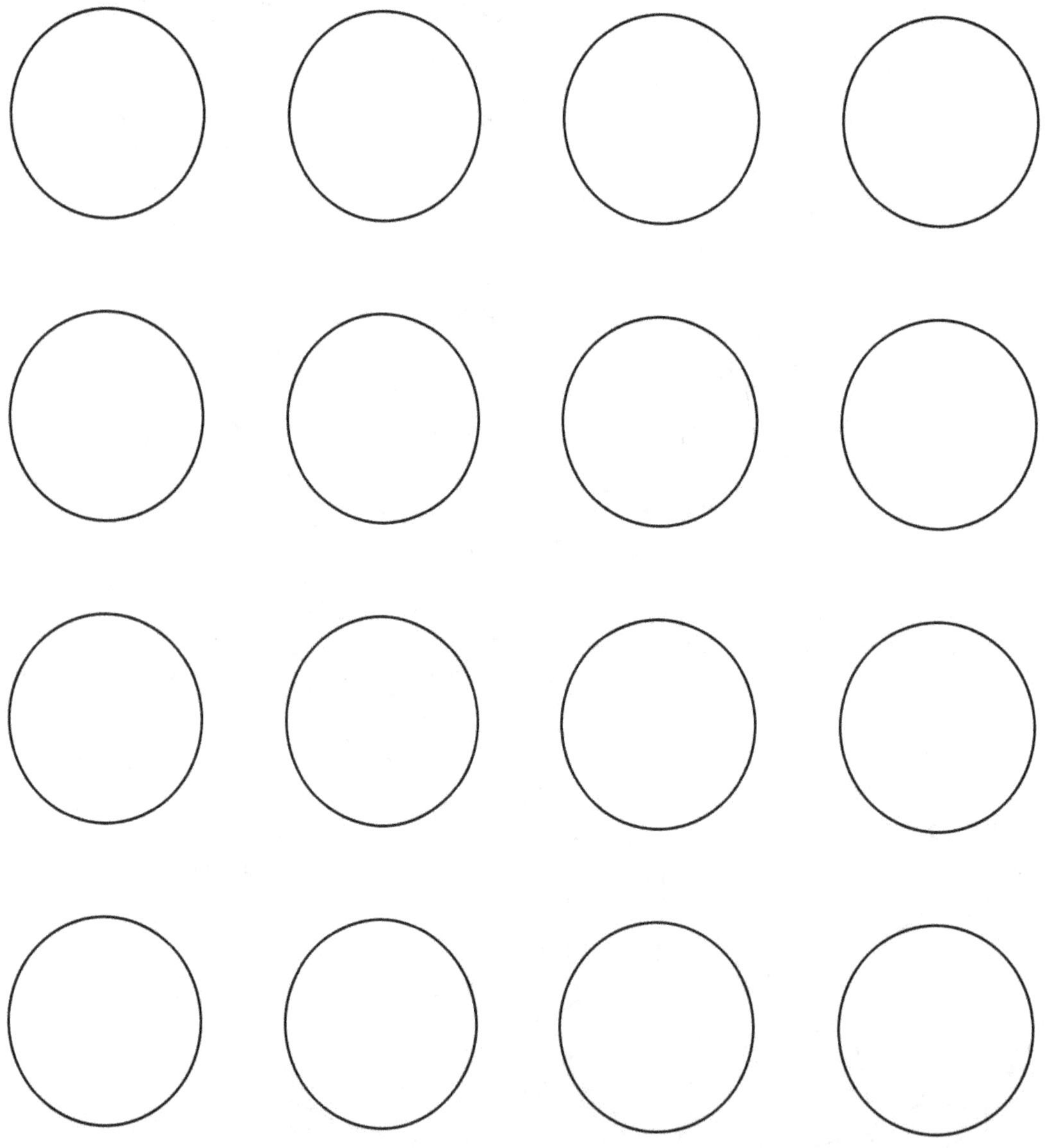

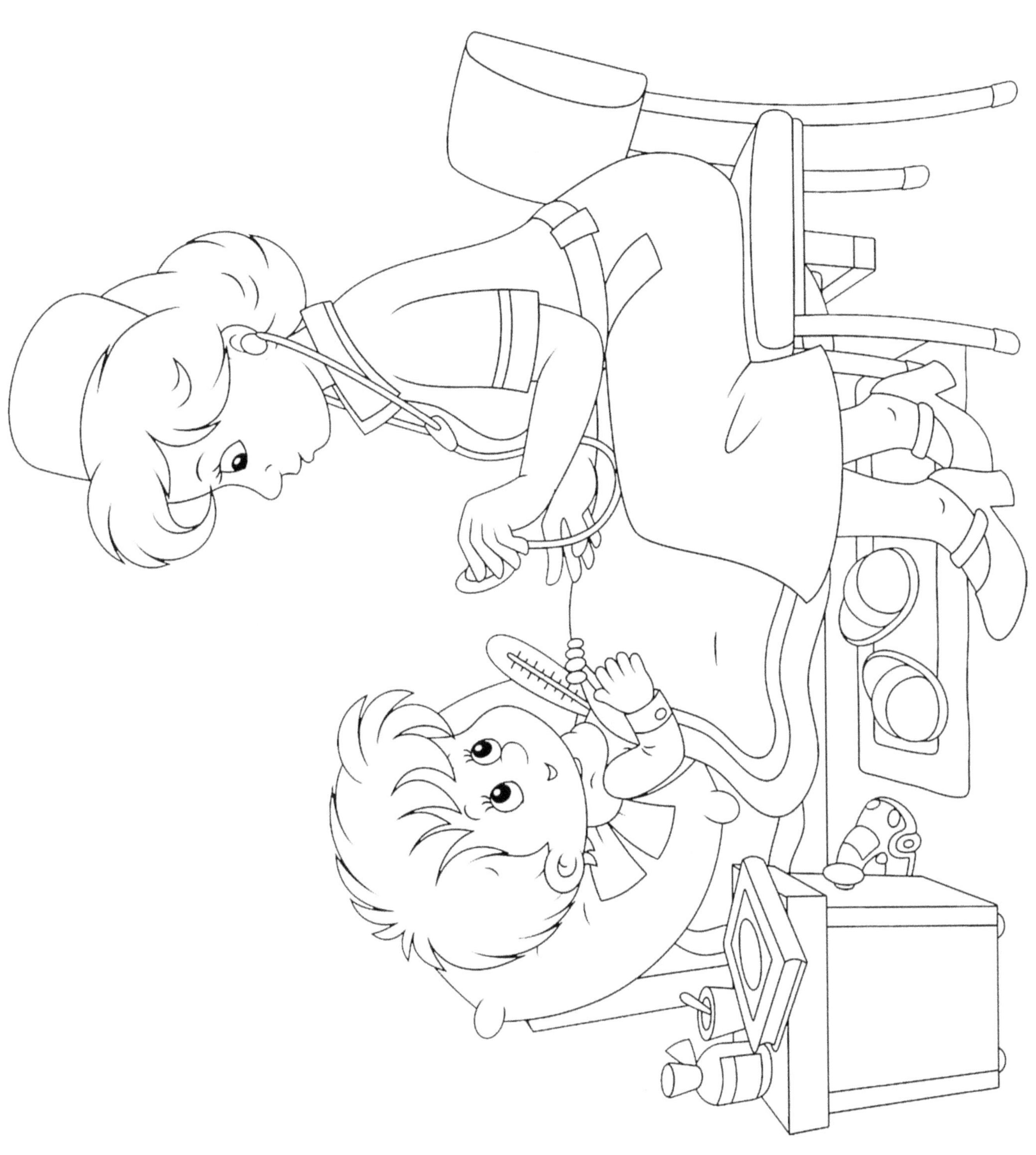

Test Your Color

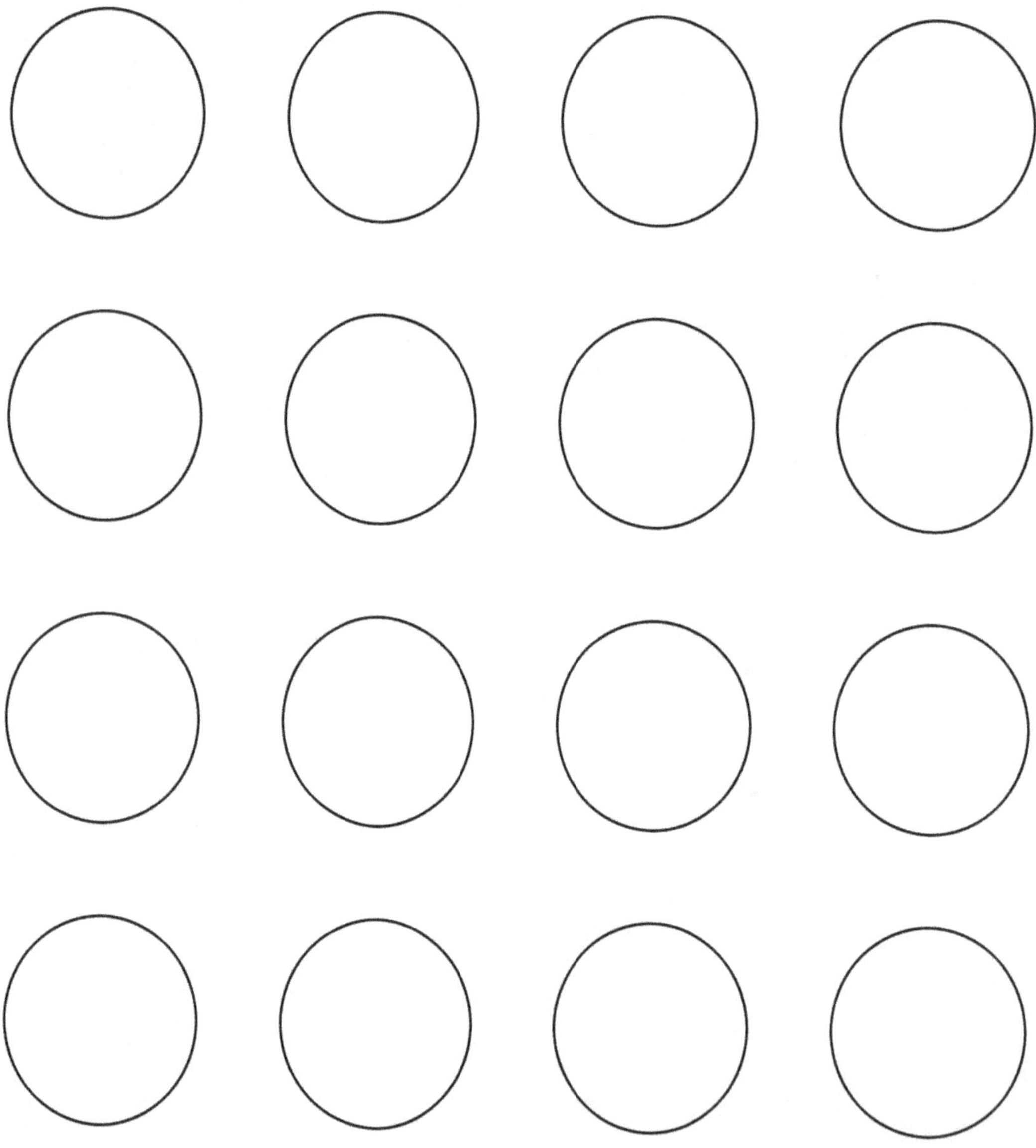

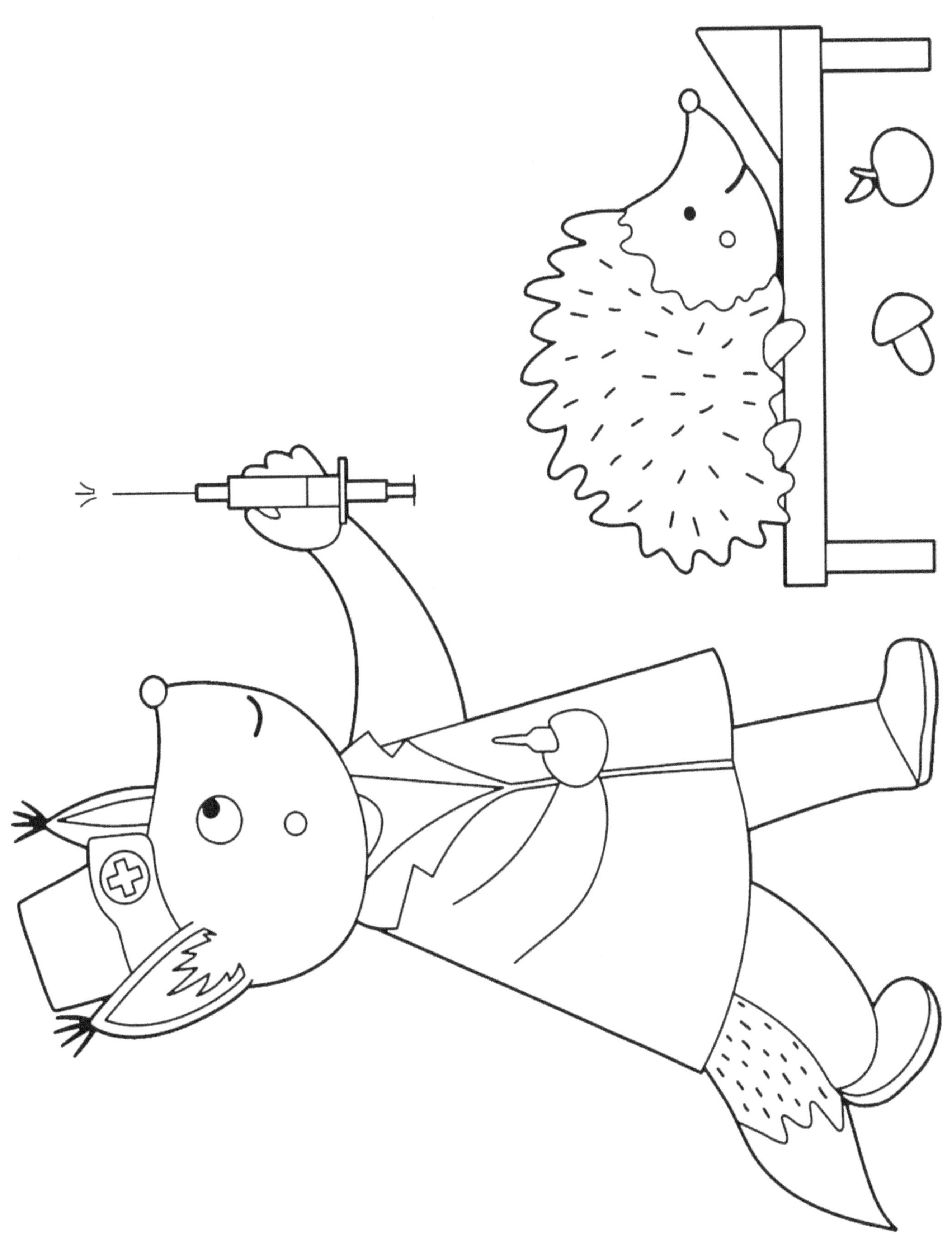

Test Your Color

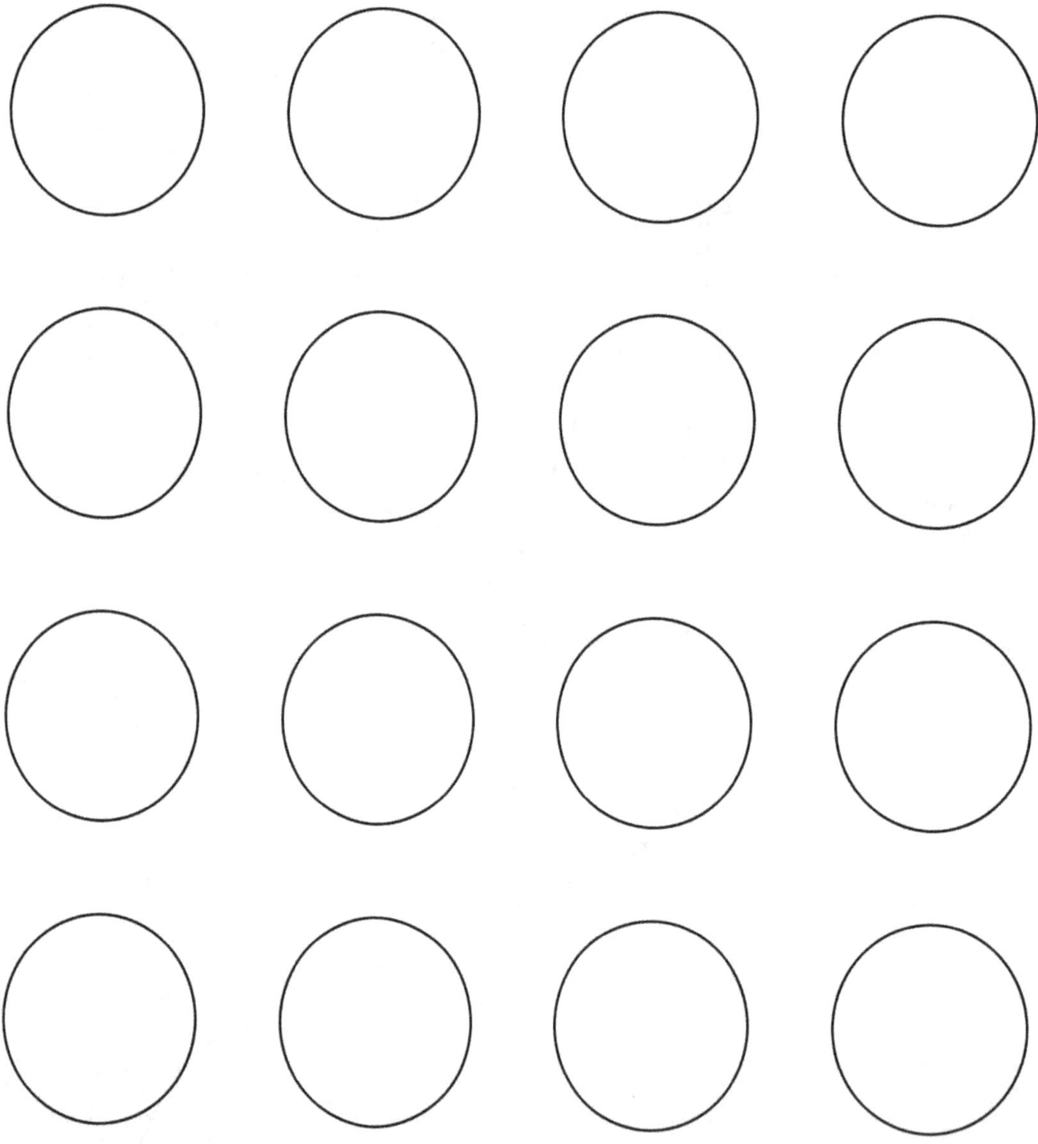

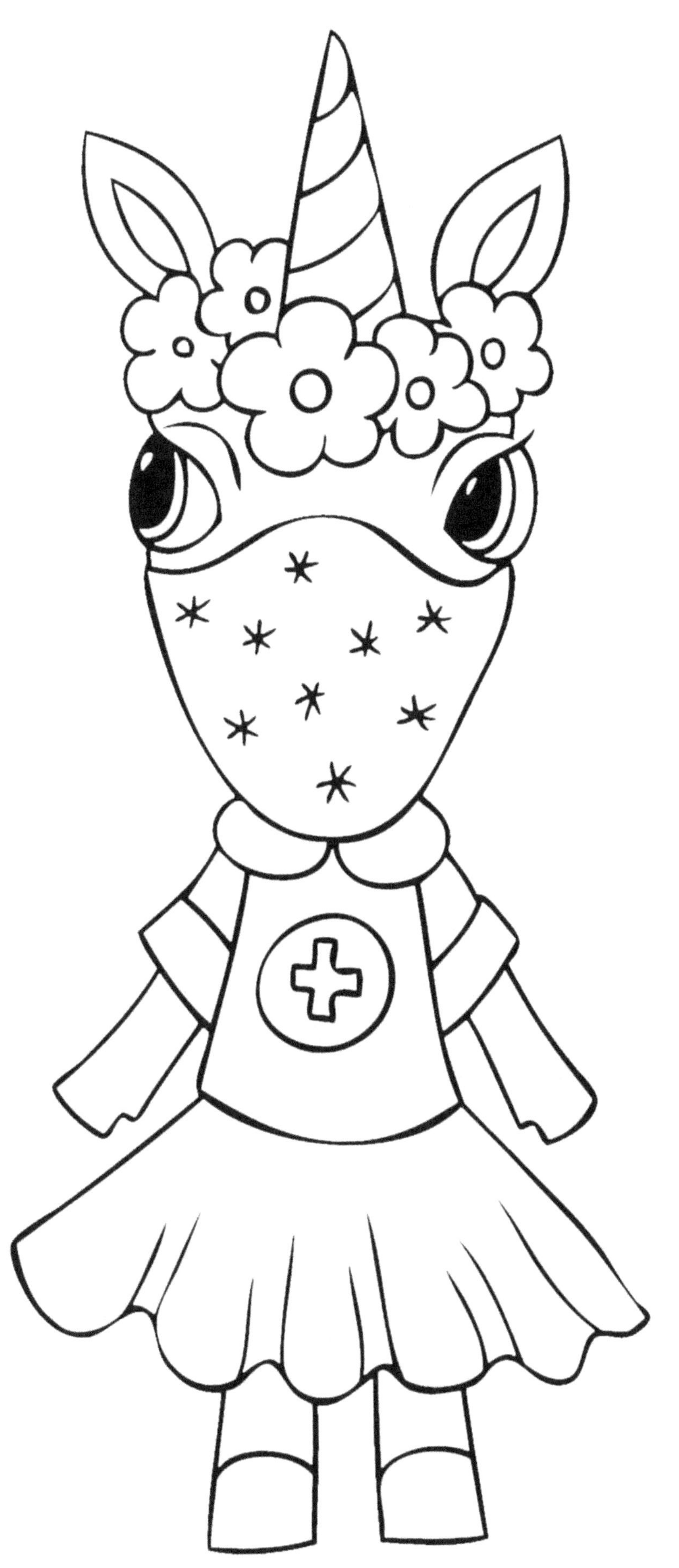

Test Your Color

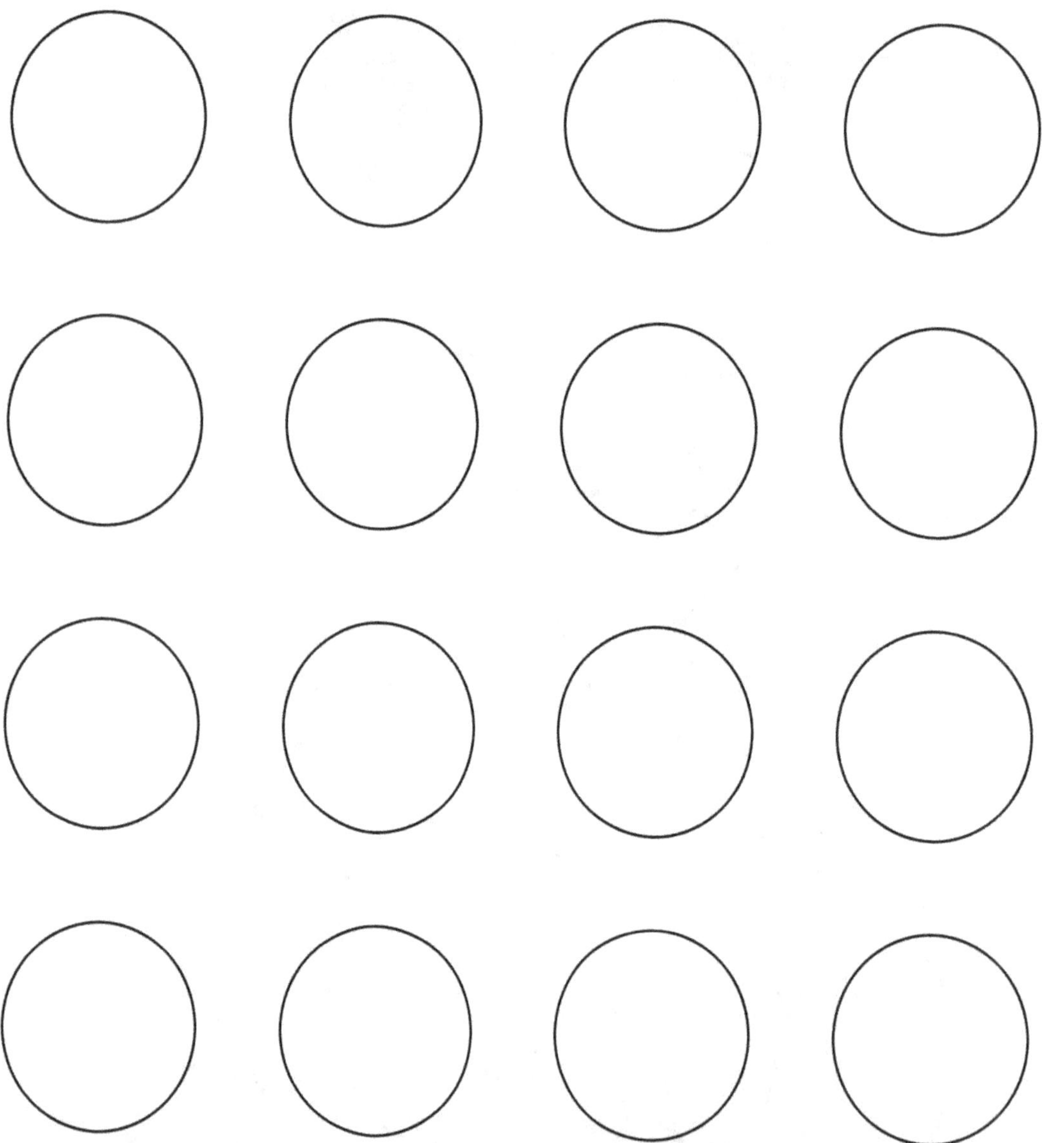

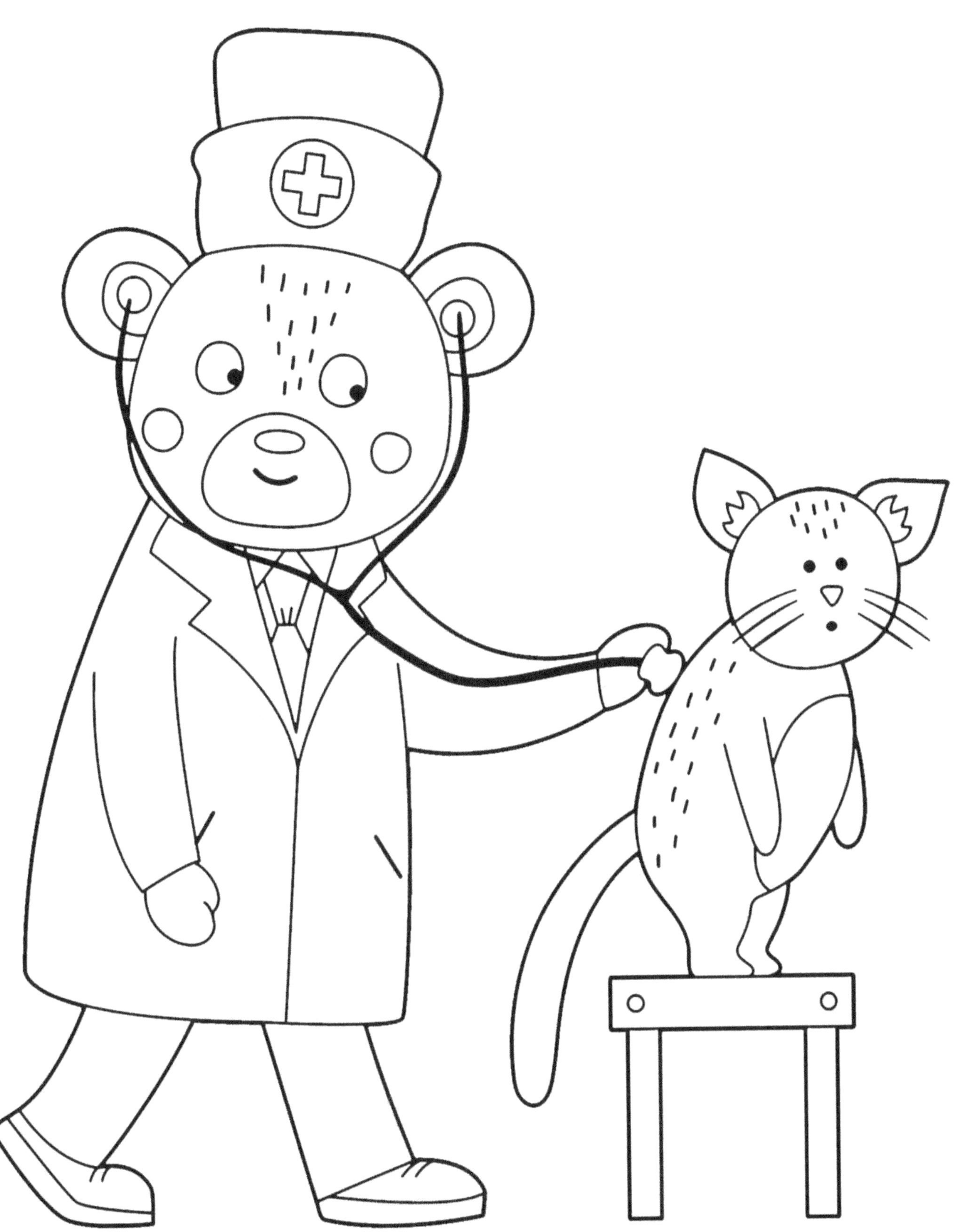

Test Your Color

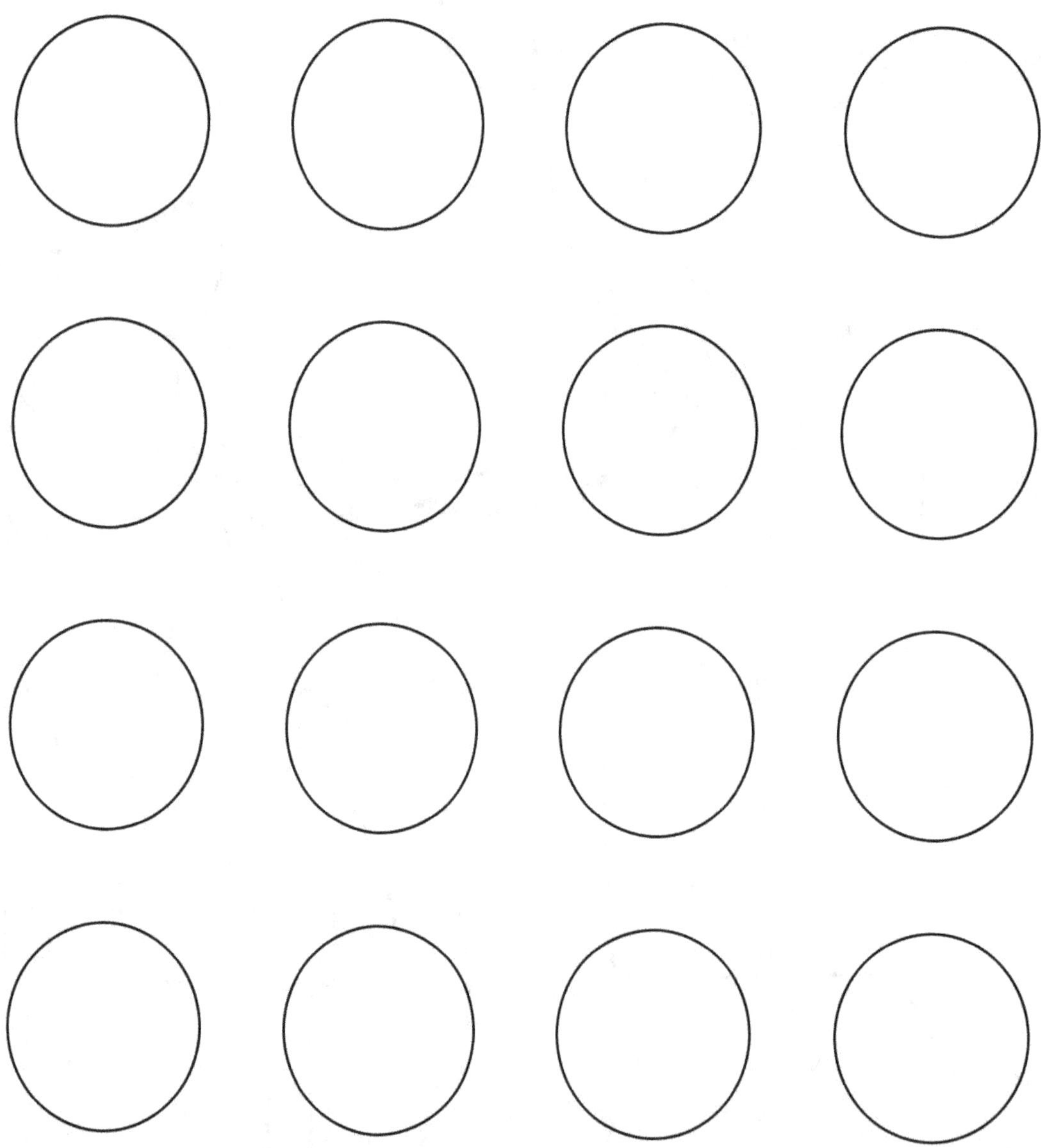

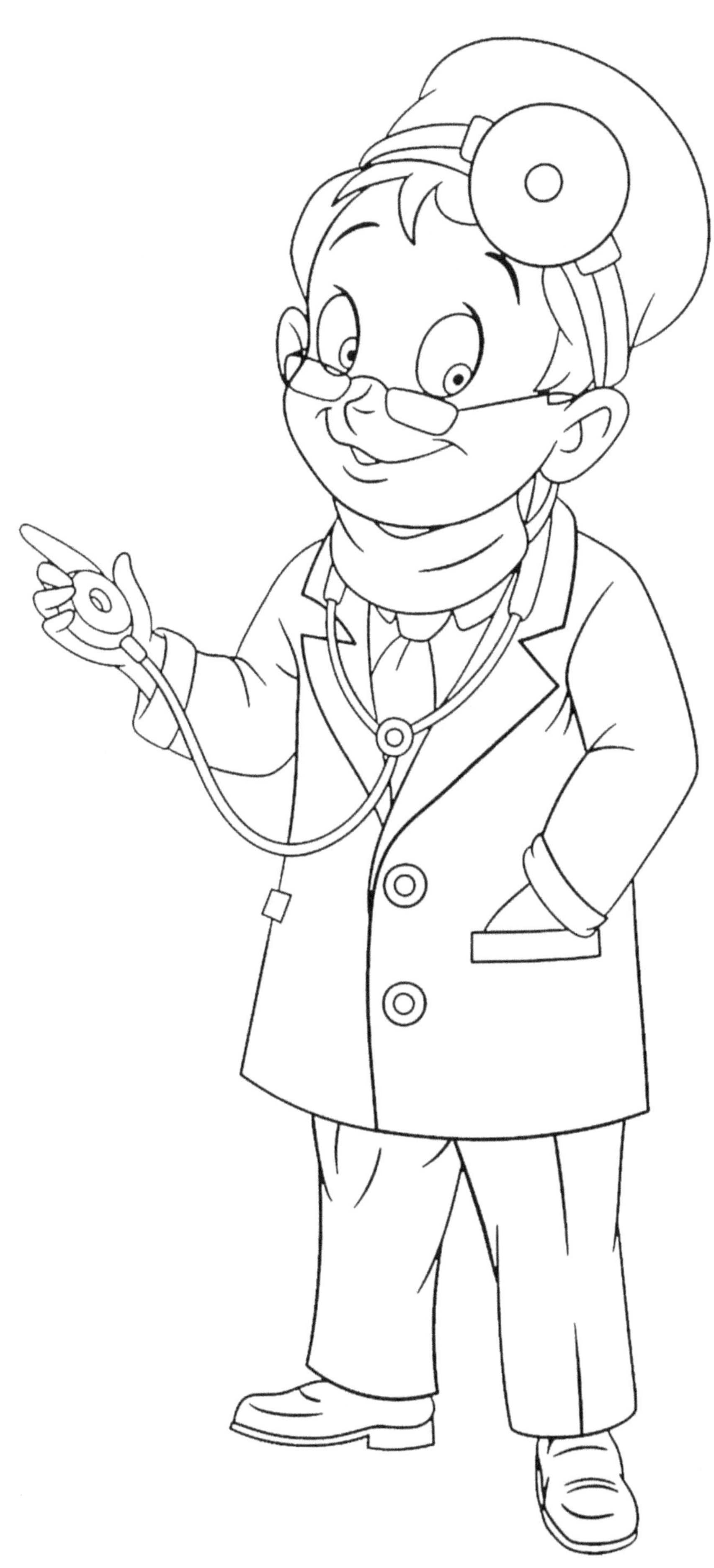

Test Your Color

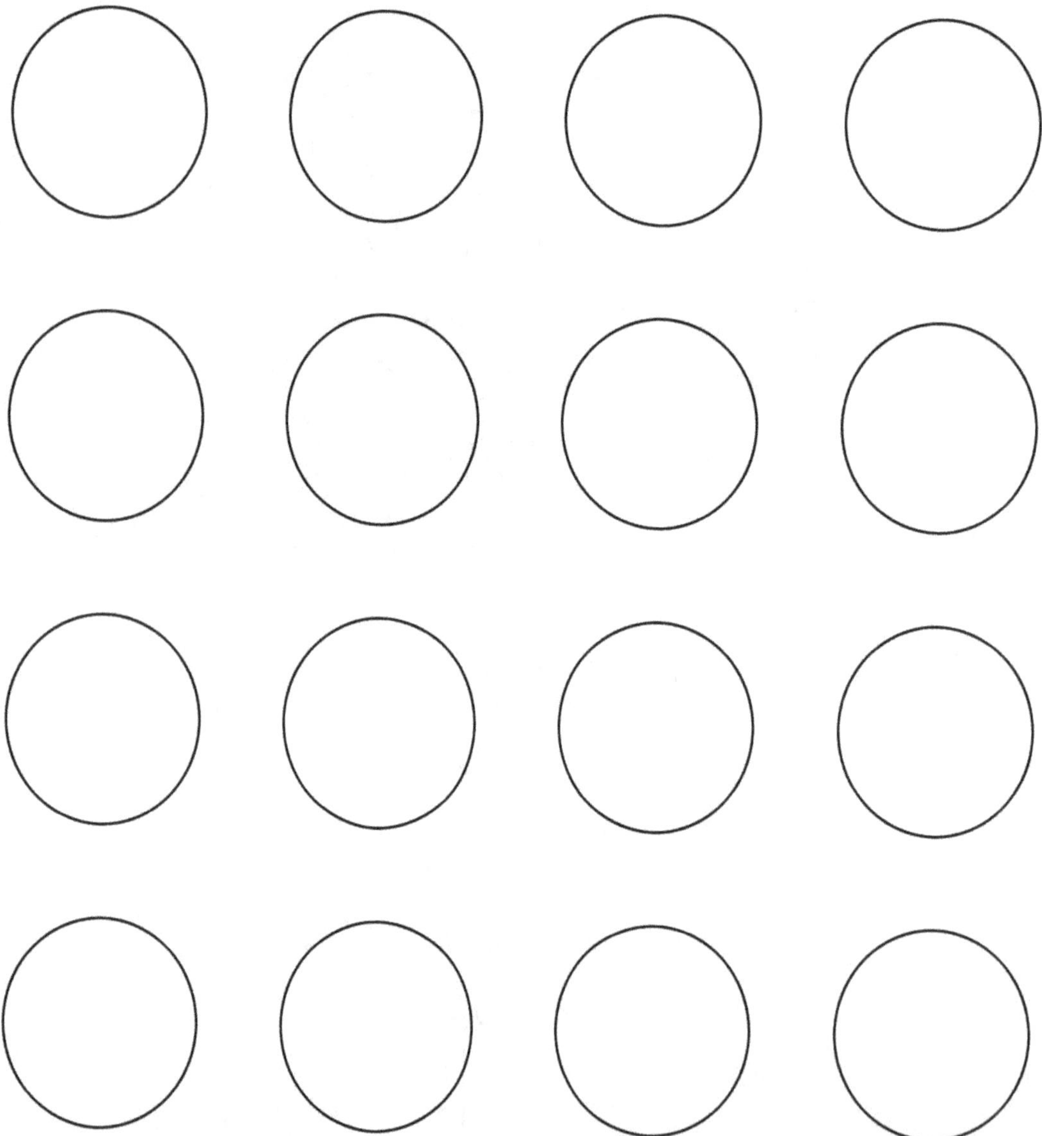

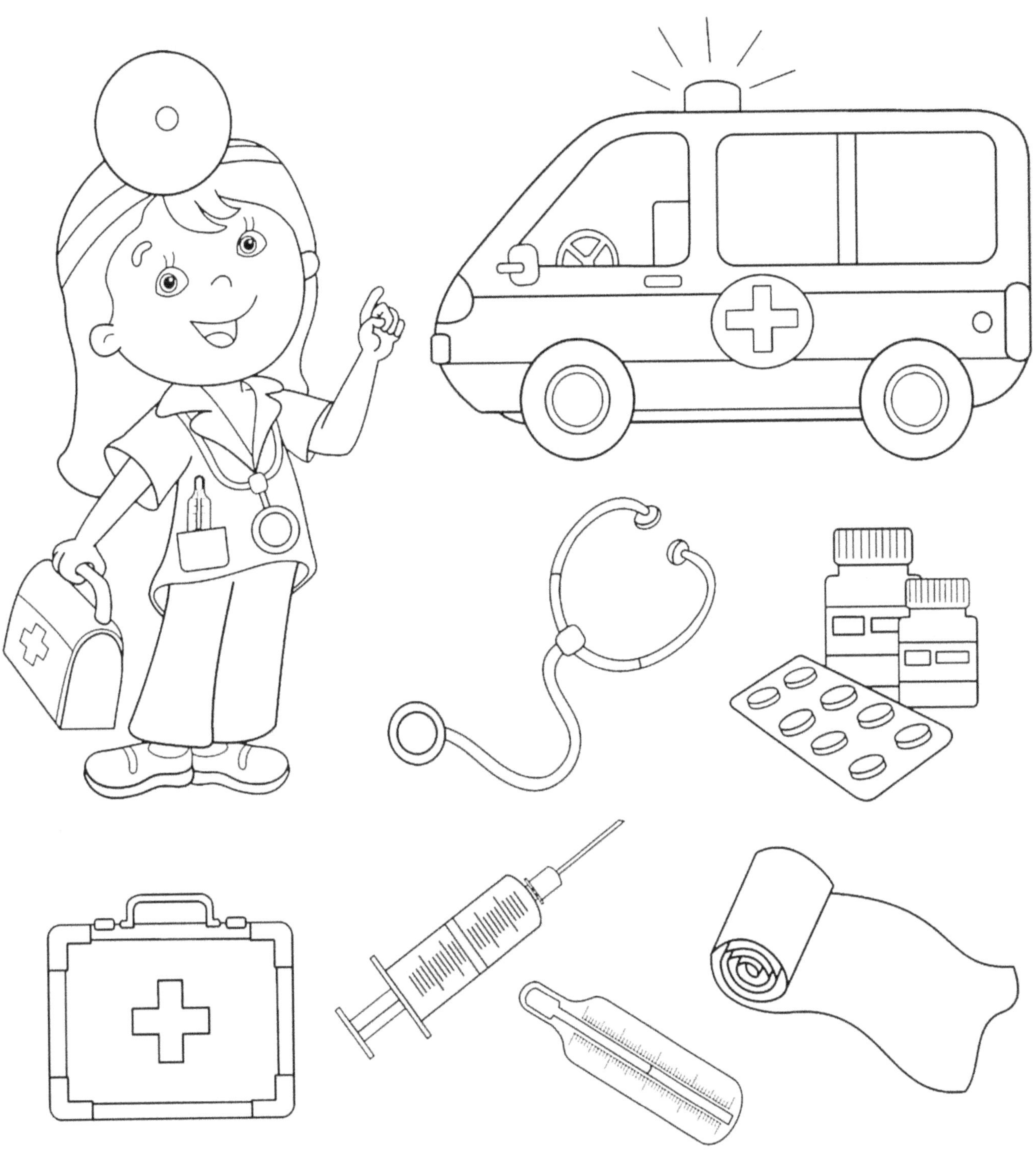

Test Your Color

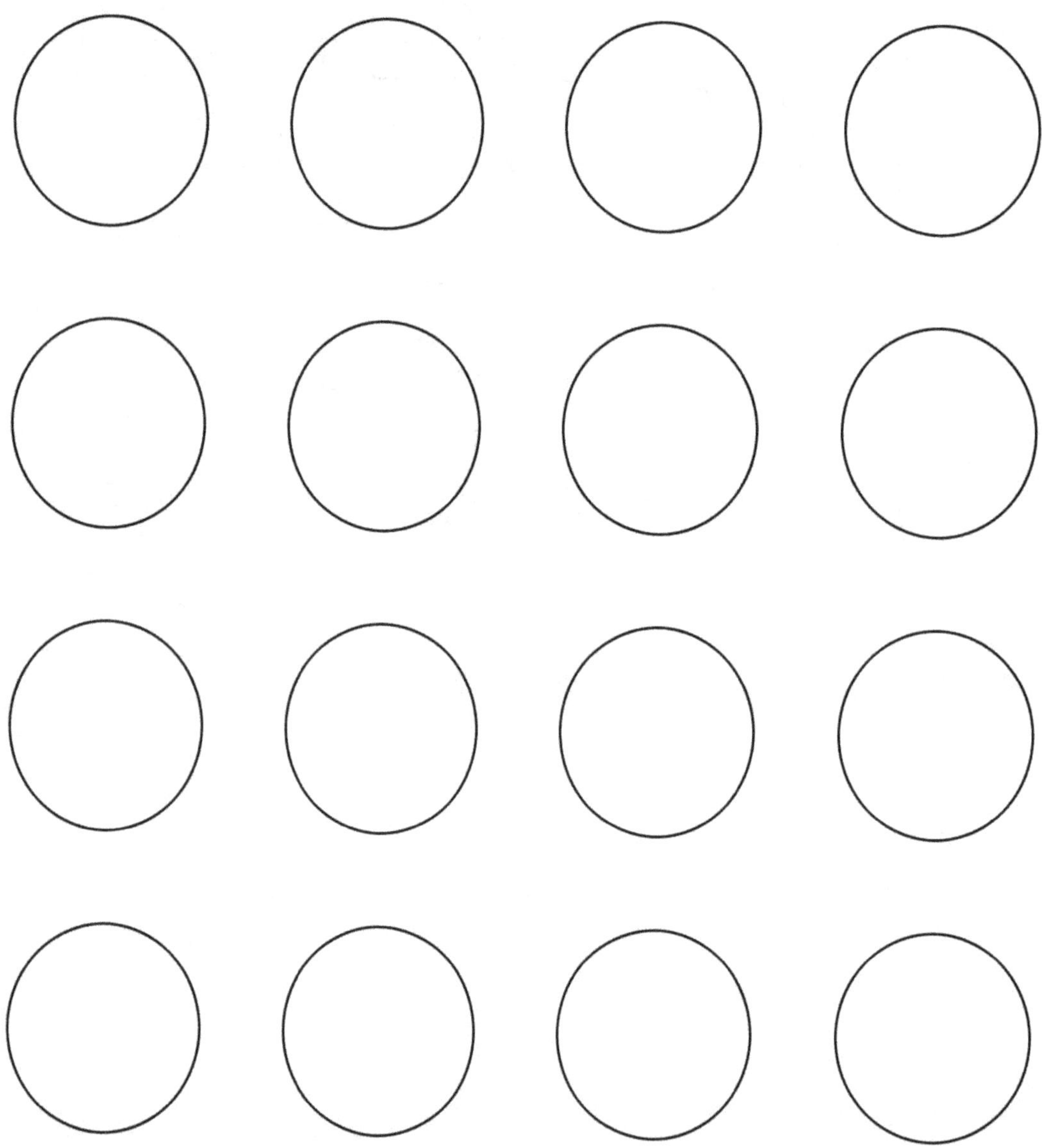

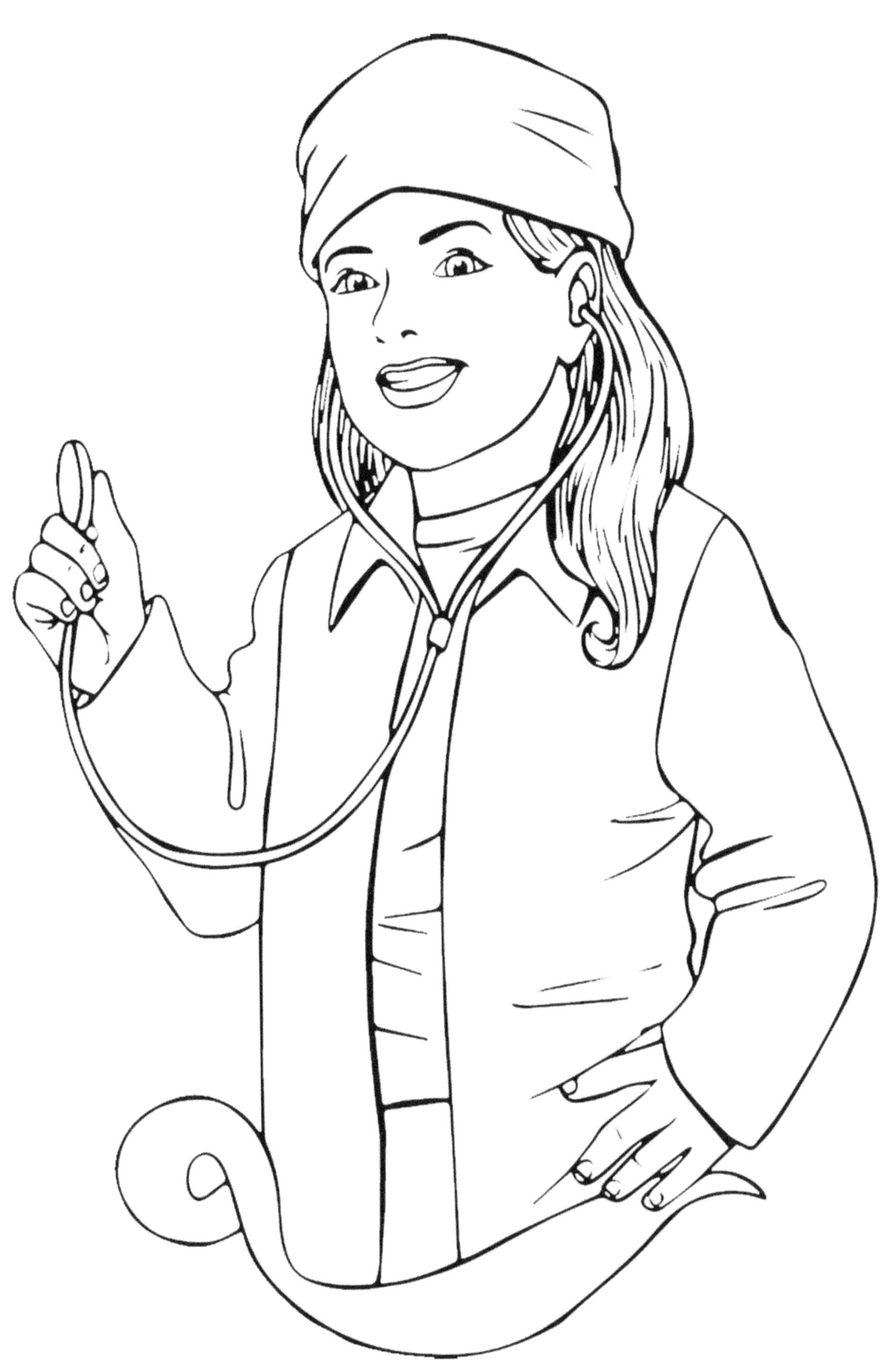

Test Your Color

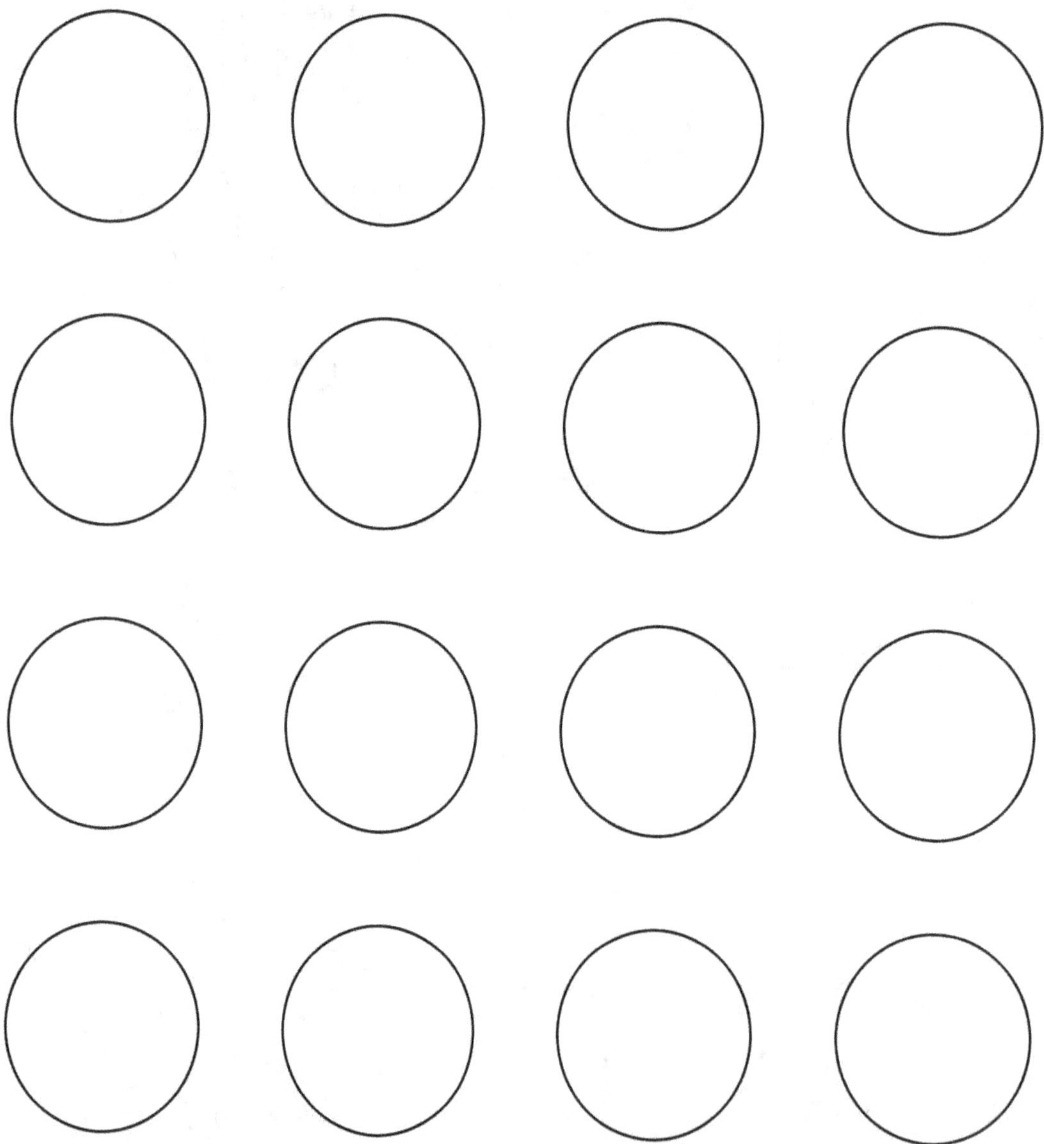

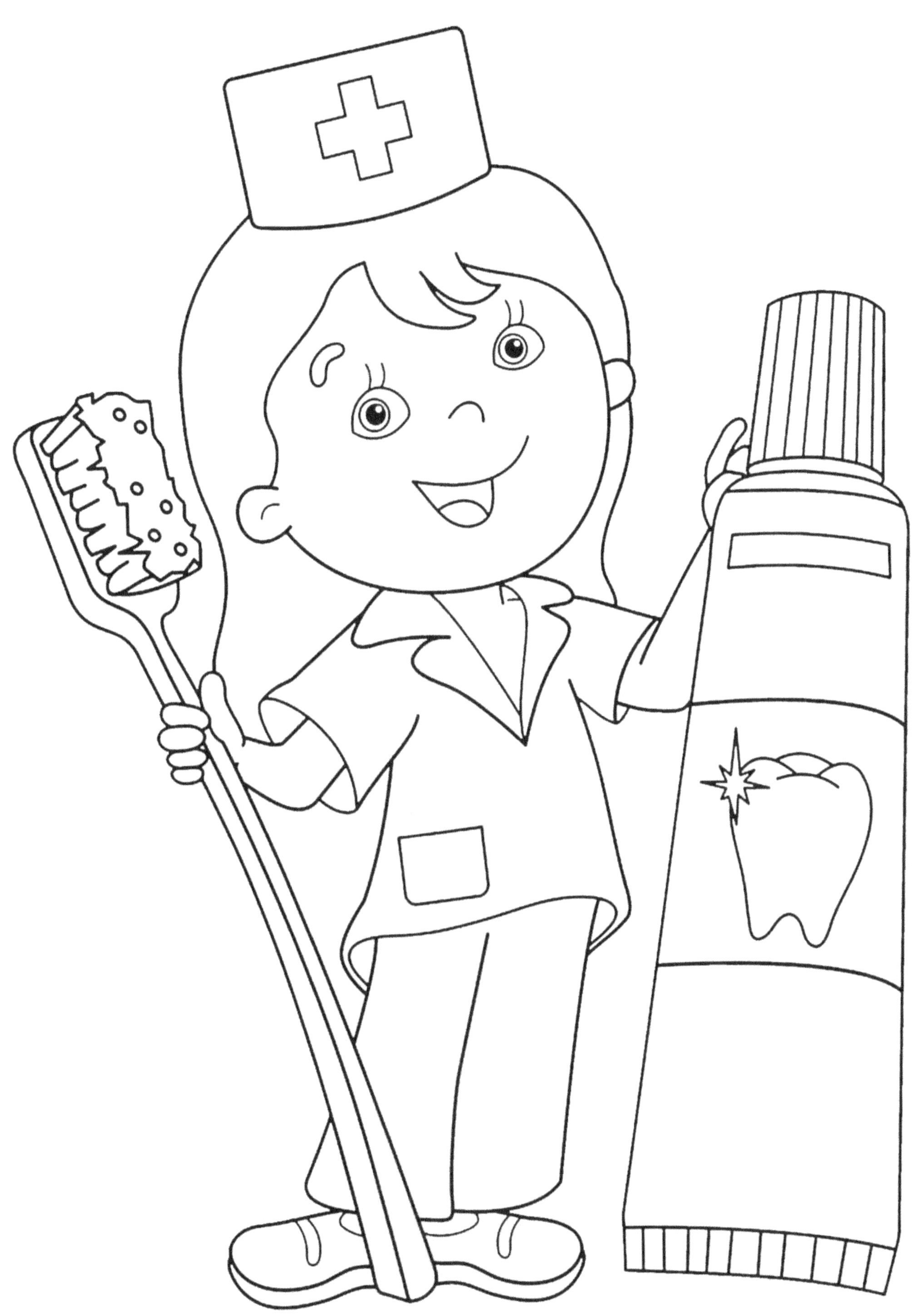

Test Your Color

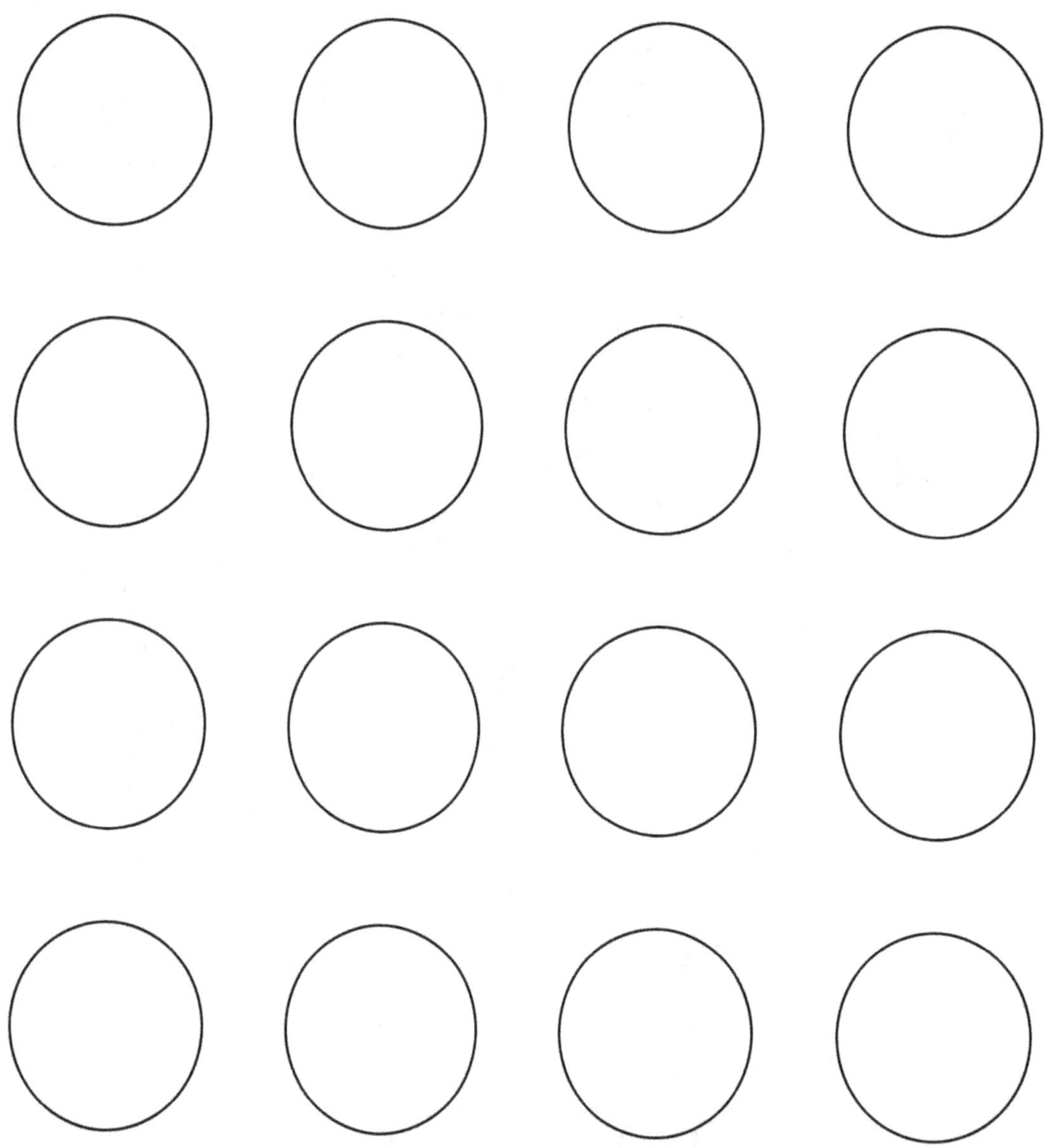

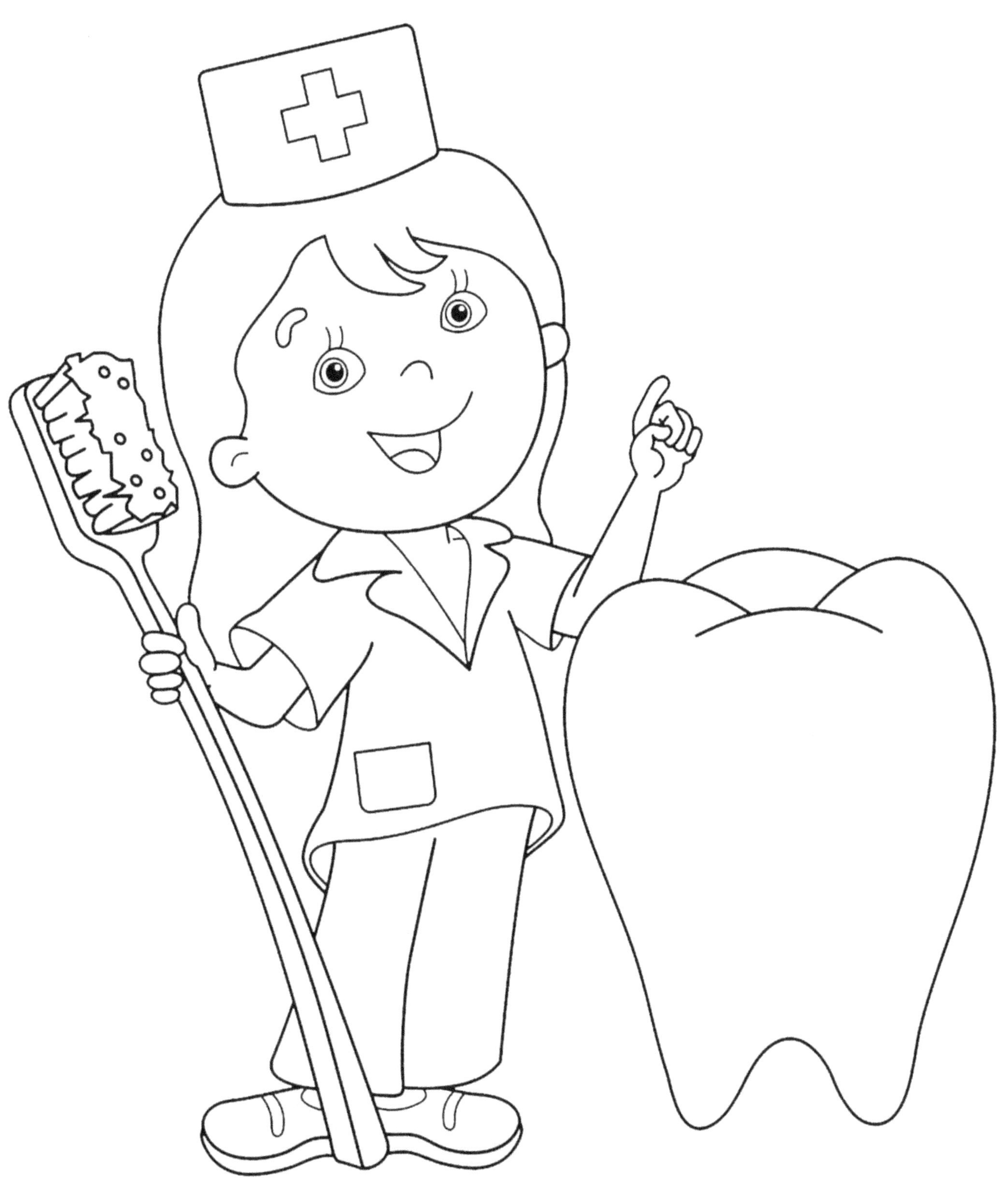

Test Your Color

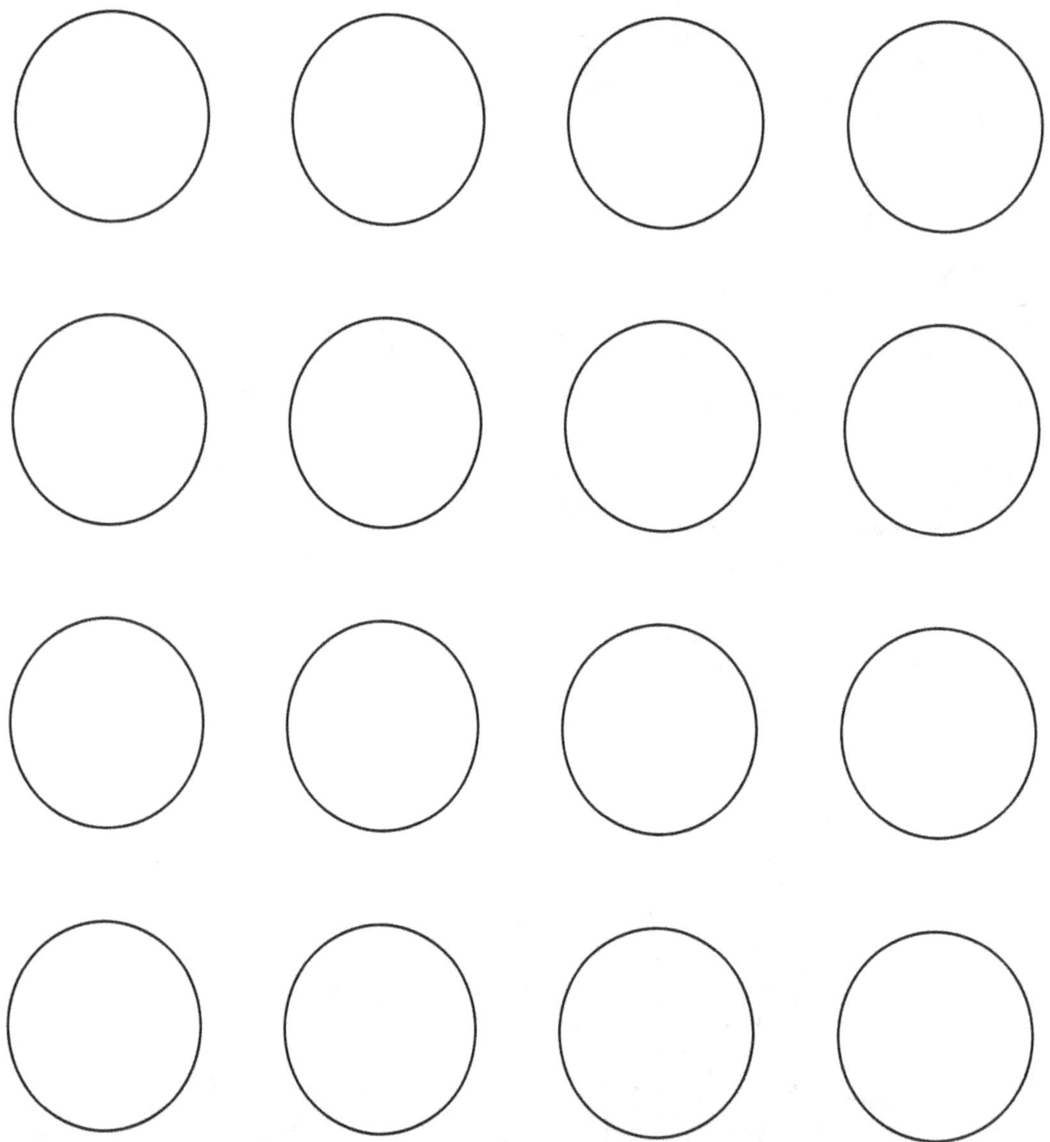

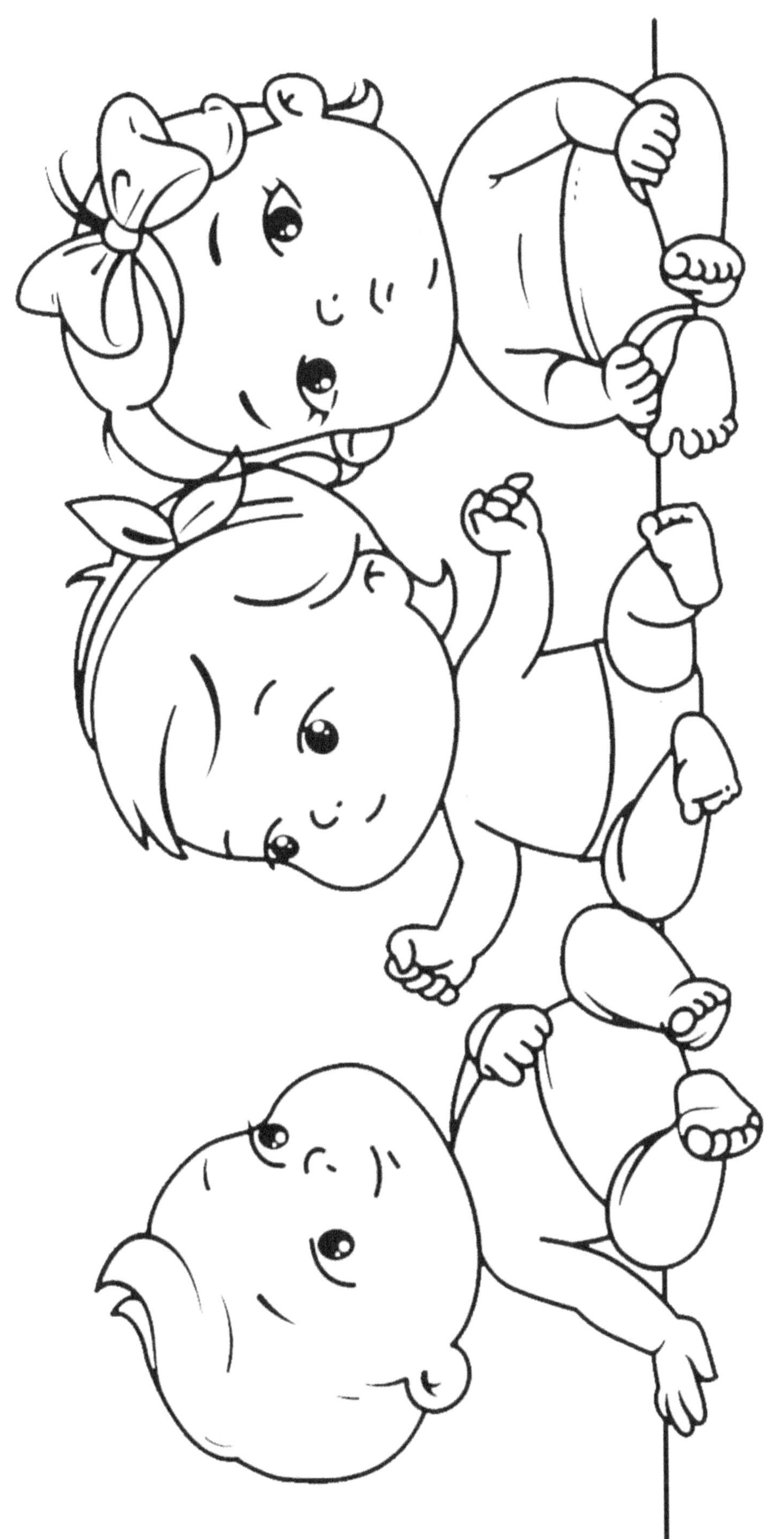

Test Your Color

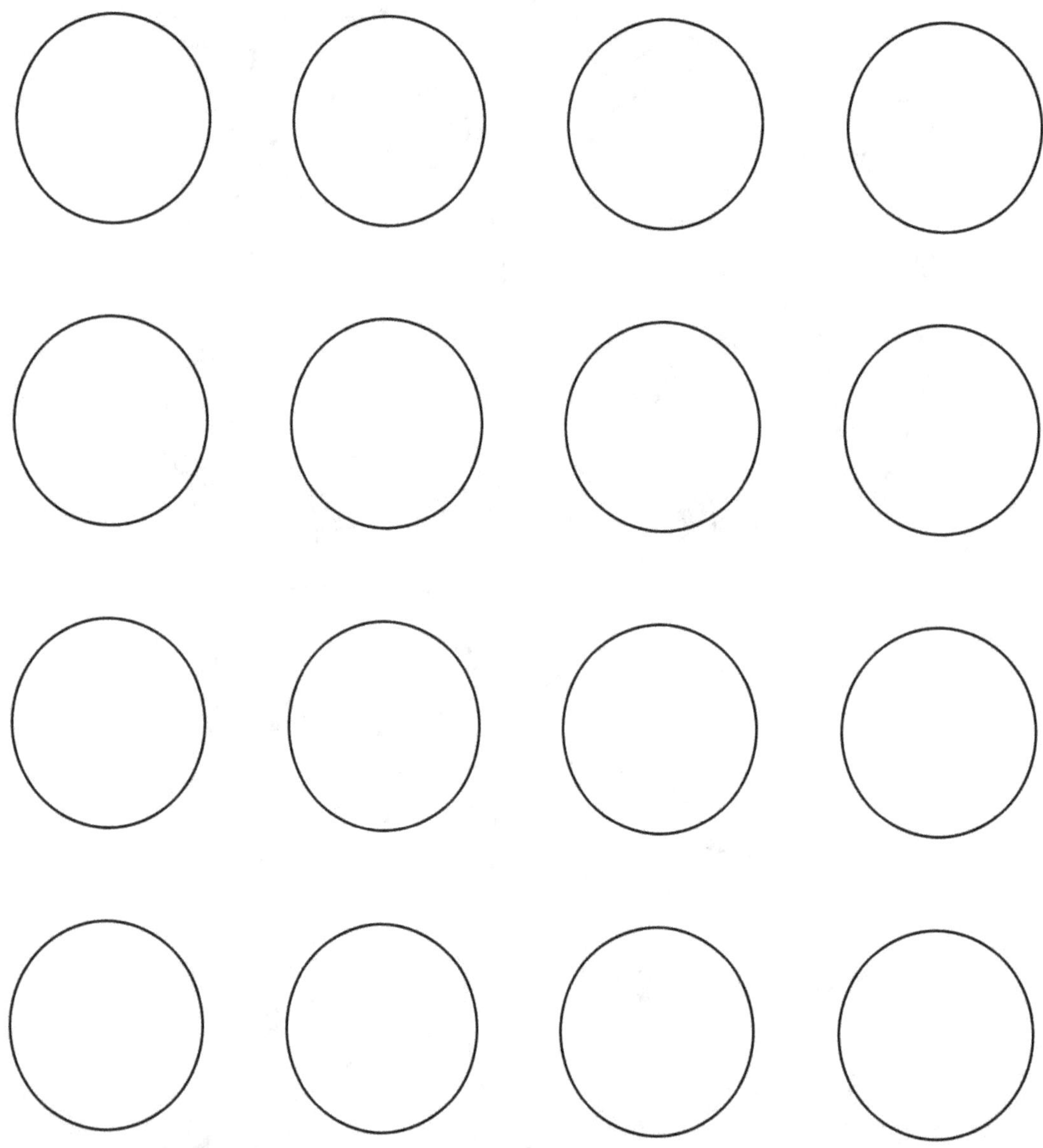